Chronic Pain the Drug-free Way

Phil Sizer started his career in the gold bullion world. In time he discovered that people were more interesting than lots of big numbers and corporate life.

He moved to Scotland with the intention of doing something creative and wholesome in a wood or up a mountain. Instead he developed an interest in stress, health and wellbeing. This ultimately led him to the world of pain management where he has worked for the last 20 years.

Phil has a passion for bringing the topics of pain management to life. He has a rare ability to work interactively with groups combining discussion with stories, metaphors and humour, so that hard-to-grasp ideas come alive.

He combines his own approach with ideas from important therapeutic approaches including: CBT (Cognitive-behavioural Therapy), Mindfulness, ACT (Acceptance and Commitment Therapy), Solution-focused therapy, Positive Psychology, Coaching and Relaxation. Unusually he also brings a background in Philosophy to the mix. This all creates a refreshing, credible approach to the work that has helped many people in thousands of sessions.

Originally from the Cambridge area, he now lives near Edinburgh with his wife Gill and their eccentric cats Noggin and Pogel.

Overcoming Common Problems Series

Selected titles

Overcoming Common Problems Series

Overcoming Common Problems Series

Overcoming Fear with Mindfulness
Deborah Ward

Overcoming Gambling: A guide for problem and compulsive gamblers
Philip Mawer

Overcoming Jealousy
Dr Windy Dryden

Overcoming Low Self-esteem with Mindfulness
Deborah Ward

Overcoming Stress
Professor Robert Bor, Dr Carina Eriksen and Dr Sara Chaudry

Overcoming Worry and Anxiety: Self-help strategies that work
Dr Jerry Kennard

The Pain Management Handbook: Your personal guide
Neville Shone

Parenting Your Disabled Child: The first three years
Margaret Barrett

Post-Traumatic Stress Disorder: Recovery after accident and disaster
Professor Kevin Gournay

Reducing Your Risk of Dementia
Dr Tom Smith

The Self-esteem Journal
Alison Waines

Sleep Better: The science and the myths
Professor Graham Law and Dr Shane Pascoe

Stress-related Illness
Dr Tim Cantopher

The Stroke Survival Guide
Mark Greener

Taming the Beast Within: Understanding personality disorder
Professor Peter Tyrer

Ten Steps to Positive Living
Dr Windy Dryden

Therapy Pets: A guide
Jill Eckersley

Toxic People: Dealing with dysfunctional relationships
Dr Tim Cantopher

Treat Your Own Knees
Jim Johnson

Treating Arthritis: The drug-free way
Margaret Hills and Christine Horner

Treating Arthritis: More ways to a drug-free life
Margaret Hills

Treating Arthritis: The supplements guide
Julia Davies

Treating Arthritis Diet Book
Margaret Hills

Treating Arthritis Exercise Book
Margaret Hills and Janet Horwood

Understanding High Blood Pressure
Dr Shahid Aziz and Dr Zara Aziz

Understanding Hoarding
Jo Cooke

Understanding Obsessions and Compulsions
Dr Frank Tallis

Vertigo and Dizziness
Jaydip Ray

Wellbeing: Body confidence, health and happiness
Emma Woolf

When Someone You Love Has Dementia
Susan Elliot-Wright

When Someone You Love Has Depression: A handbook for family and friends
Barbara Baker

The Whole Person Recovery Handbook
Emma Drew

Your Guide for the Cancer Journey: Cancer and its treatment
Mark Greener

Lists of titles in the Mindful Way and Sheldon Short Guides series are also available from Sheldon Press.

Overcoming Common Problems

Chronic Pain the Drug-free Way

PHIL SIZER

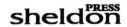
sheldon PRESS

First published in Great Britain in 2019 by Sheldon Press, an imprint of
John Murray Press. An Hachette UK company.

A CIP catalogue record for this title is available from the British Library

Paperback: 978 1 84709 479 7
eBook: 978 1 84709 480 3

Typeset by Fakenham Prepress Solutions, Fakenham, Norfolk NR21 8NL
Printed and bound in Great Britain by Clays Ltd, Elcograf S.p.A

John Murray Learning policy is to use papers that are natural, renewable
and recyclable products and made from wood grown in sustainable
forests. The logging and manufacturing processes are expected to
conform to the environmental regulations of the country of origin.

Sheldon Press
Carmelite House
50 Victoria Embankment
London EC4Y 0DZ
www.sheldonpress.co.uk

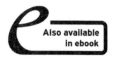

Contents

To Gill and my parents, Janet and Gerald

Foreword

First and foremost, I am delighted that Phil Sizer, our lead trainer at Pain Association Scotland, has been given the opportunity to write about the self-management skills and strategies he delivers with great passion each day to all those burdened with chronic pain. I am so glad that he is now sharing his knowledge here. I would also like to thank Neville Shone for facilitating the opportunity for Phil to produce this book. For many years, Neville has provided significant input to the work of the Association and continues to support this by being one of our valued patrons.

Chronic pain is a major individual, societal and economic burden. For most individuals with chronic pain, it is not about the length of time they have had the pain, but about the loss of function, loss of identity, loss of mental health and, indeed, for many, loss of hope (Eccleston, 2011, 2016). We see this every day in our work. People are often told by clinicians, 'There is nothing more we can do for you', but, although that may be true medically, it is not true of more general strategies. Remember, however, that no one is saying the journey will be easy or free from challenges.

The work of the Association is delivered through intensive self-management courses and local monthly self-management group meetings throughout Scotland, Northumbria and North Wales. Our service delivery is person centred and based on a biopsychosocial model. It is not just about the pain but, rather, the focus is on dealing with pain in the wider context of life, health and well-being. It is about looking at the impact that everyday events have on living with this long-term condition – the impact on relationships, work and social life, the effect of medicines and so on, and we provide a combination of learning and education with normalization and peer support. This helps our clients become less dependent on medical help and, instead, to engage realistically with ideas, discuss them, hear from those who have made progress, support those who are struggling and thereby integrate self-management into their everyday lives. Indeed, our self-management education and learning programmes are designed to meet this need and create a very can-do approach.

One of the mechanisms responsible for the improvements in health shown by those attending self-management programmes is self-efficacy. Self-management support has been defined as 'increasing the capacity, confidence and efficacy of the individual'. The outcomes from our intensive courses and groups demonstrate that self-efficacy is increased and coping skills are maintained more effectively by those who go on to attend the monthly group meetings. Chronic pain and its impact cannot be ignored – it is a national priority, which is why the Association has continued to develop a valuable service through collaborative working relationships with respective National Health Service Boards and our service users.

Living from day to day with chronic pain can often be viewed as, in essence, dealing with a sense of grief – individuals' grief for the person they once were and what they could once do within their work, social or family life. One difficulty is that the implications of living with this pain are often not visible to the outside world, which frequently creates a lack of understanding. On reading the book, you will very quickly see that your pain *is* believed, even though it may be invisible.

Sensitivity to pain is not a sign of weakness, and there is no reason to feel shame or guilt if pain appears to affect you more than it does other people. Many factors contribute to how disruptive pain is for us as individuals and many of these factors are out of our control.

As no two people have the same experience, even if they have the same disease or diagnosis, the aim of this book is to help you take back control of your pain. Self-management is not easy; it is a journey and, unfortunately, chronic pain will not follow your plans – instead, it will change them quite significantly. Reading this book will, however, help you to look at what you *can* do, despite the pain, and be the change you want to see.

The final word from me should be a health warning: as you read this book, be prepared to question yourself over the difficulties of managing and living with this long-term condition, but also trust in the empowerment you experience as you begin to take back control rather than have the pain control you.

Sonia Cottom
Director, Pain Association Scotland

Note to the reader

This is not a medical book and is not intended to replace advice from your doctor. Consult your pharmacist or doctor if you have any worries or concerns about your health, and if you think you might need medical help.

Introduction

'Chronic pain' is a medical term that simply means long-term pain. The 'chronic' bit comes from the Greek word for time – *chronos* – and you will know all too well what 'pain' is.

The medical definition of pain is that it is 'an unpleasant sensory and emotional experience'. That means there's 'ouch' and a feeling of upset at the same time. This, of course, understates it, but that definition covers all pain. For example, if you hit your thumb with a hammer, it throbs and you may swear. In theory, pain is there to protect us, alert us to damage in the body and help stop us hitting our thumb with a hammer, but when there is a long-term condition, pain is not so useful. Many different conditions are associated with chronic pain, but regardless of the condition, and even if you do not have a diagnosis, the experience of living with pain in the long term is universally the same – well, quite simply, it's a pain!

There are far more people living with chronic pain than you would think – it's roughly the same as the number of white cars on the road (19 per cent). It is an enormous health and social welfare problem that often goes unnoticed because people look well, feel stigmatized and don't want to talk about it. Chronic pain is notoriously hard to treat medically and has a huge impact on quality of life and well-being. Understandably, people often feel abandoned, isolated, helpless and hopeless.

The difficulty is that everyone is clamouring for more medical help. Of course, medical help is important to a point, but chronic pain is far more than just a medical condition. The focus on clinical approaches, such as painkilling tablets, injections of painkillers or anti-inflammatory medicines, and operations often means that wider issues, such as what is happening in your daily life, are ignored.

Obviously, we all want a cure for chronic pain, but medical professionals rightly say that a cure is unlikely, and this can be hard to accept. They also say that drugs often do not work as well as we hope and they always have side effects. They may say, 'You need to manage it yourself', but this is not something anyone wants to hear.

I have met thousands of people who have been told, 'I'm sorry, there's nothing more we can do for you.' This statement can go off like a bomb in someone's life. People often feel abandoned and fear that they are now on the scrapheap, but it doesn't mean that all hope is lost: it just means that, from a *medical* point of view, no more can be done. If you have been told this or this news is coming, or you don't want to wait, then this book is for you.

One reason chronic pain is a nuisance is because pain levels vary day to day, often for no apparent reason. It's therefore hard to plan ahead and easy to fall into the trap of going flat out whenever pain lets you, then crashing afterwards – flat out to flat out. This cycle of overactivity and forced rest, of booming and then busting, is very stressful. Stress and pain can feed off each other and create an unpleasant set of repeating vicious cycles. It's no surprise, then, that chronic pain can take over your life. Everything in the day can be dictated by a person's pain level, which can eclipse the things that makes them feel happy and fulfilled.

Looking beyond the pain itself, people often face many challenges that make a difficult situation worse. Stress, unemployment, anxiety, sleeplessness and low mood are all examples of the impact that a change in health can have, adding further limitations that just add to the already difficult situation caused by chronic pain. Dealing with those challenges is often the way to improve life, despite chronic pain. The approach outlined in this book is not a cure, but it does offer a way forward that is especially important if we are realistic and see progress in terms of improving the situation. It is aimed to help you manage and cope with your condition yourself rather than being wholly dependent on medical help.

This approach is often called 'self'-management because it's all about what you, and only you, can change. I am not, of course, suggesting that you start operating on yourself, creating your own potions or ignoring your doctor's advice; instead, I am suggesting that anything you can do to improve your pain, your life or both is vitally important, and the sooner you do it, the better.

Defining progress solely in terms of pain level is a hard taskmaster, especially when the pain is not showing much change. On one course I led, a tuba player (and you don't get many of those) kept saying to me, 'When do we do the bit that gets rid of the pain?' He was so fixated on the pain and getting rid of it that the pain was all he 'saw'. He wanted solutions that would make his pain disappear instantly. His view was that everything was ruined by the pain, so the only solution was to get rid of it. Sadly, that meant he lacked the patience to do anything else, such as reduce his stress levels to help him defuse the pain bomb. It was a tough experience for both of us. He kept pushing and I kept disappointing him.

This book is about a longer-term, slower-burn solution that many people describe as a journey. That may sound corny, but it takes time to turn the supertanker of life around. This approach is not for everyone – or maybe it is, but how you respond to it depends on where you are on that journey. Even if you think this approach makes little sense and you cannot do it, it's a step forward in the journey. Even if you vow you cannot do any of it, at least you will know that there is an alternative way forward.

Over the time I have been doing this kind of work, I have seen many different varieties of improvement: some people go back to work, others stay in work, some get on better at home, some find benefit in relaxation or get fitter through pacing, while others learn to be kinder to themselves. Some improve their sleep pattern, others say they feel more in control. Some take up a hobby and feel happier in themselves. Some plan better; others say that they have fewer flare-ups. Some take fewer medicines so have fewer side effects, while others say they feel more at peace. Everyone, though, says that they cope better in one way or another. Some even do see an improvement in their pain.

The reality of chronic pain is that we live with it – it's not just a medical condition that can be easily cured, but something with long-term effects on life and how you experience it more generally. If we can make changes and live better with our pain, if we manage what we can and find a different way of thinking, something will improve. I hope this book will help you find ways to change your life and your thoughts so that, somehow, something will be different and, hopefully, better. Good luck!

Part 1
UNDERSTANDING

1

Changing perspective

The man who invented the total perspective vortex did so basically to annoy his wife.

Douglas Adams, *The Hitchhiker's Guide to the Galaxy*

When we have chronic pain, we tend to slip into blaming it for every problem we encounter. That's not a surprise because it grabs our attention and shouts at us all day. Look at things differently, however, and you will see many other issues that could be adding to your load. Some of these will contribute directly to the pain, while others are issues in themselves that just make life harder. Sometimes it is the indirectly connected issues, such as relationships or being believed, that have the biggest impact.

What helps with chronic pain is adopting a wide perspective. This means looking at the whole of life, not just the medical aspects. When you do this, you may see something important that has been missed. You may find a solution to one bit of the puzzle and therefore improve the whole. Depending on what you find, this could make a huge difference. It might change your pain or it might improve your life and ability to cope.

In the late 1970s, there was a children's television programme called *Worzel Gummidge*, about a scarecrow who comes to life. The bizarre bit that I remember was the scarecrow pulling off his grumpy, scary head made from a mangel-wurzel (a bit like a big turnip) and putting on another, far more charming one when he wanted to chat up the life-size fairground doll Aunt Sally. Even if you don't remember the show, hopefully you will get the point about different heads for different situations. We need to do something similar and take off our medical pain-focused head (remember the tuba player) and put on a different one that we can use to see the bigger picture. There might be other heads too that will help break old patterns of thinking, but we'll come to those later. First, we need to start seeing things differently.

When I meet people, I like to hear a bit of their story so that I can find clues to how to help them. Even a few words help. Sometimes there is an underlying situation that people do not think is relevant to their health. I hear many medically-related bits of information, but with my Worzel head on, what I'm really listening out for are stress and lifestyle issues. Major issues often hide in plain sight. They can be so close to us that we don't see them – a bit like when all the children shout, 'It's behind you' at a Christmas pantomime. In real life, if we are up to our necks in our situation, if our stress level is high, we can be so focused on a particular situation that we cannot see beyond it.

A lovely lady in Northumbria came to see me because her pain was 'going haywire', all this on top of the fact that her husband of 57 years had just died. 'It's the last thing I need right now', she said. She had been to the doctor repeatedly and had had everything 'checked out', but the pain still remained strong. When we spoke, I suggested that perhaps her bereavement would explain why her pain was worse. She replied, 'That's so obvious, I don't know why I didn't think of it', but at the time she was probably too upset to make the connection. Together, we looked at the next best step for her, which was bereavement counselling.

Sometimes we don't see things because we don't know they are causing difficulty. One grumpy lady folded her arms crossly and exclaimed, 'Nothing you've said has worked – my pain is still bad and I still can't sleep.' When we talked about why this might be, she admitted that she drank at least 25 cups of coffee a day. I suggested that she reduce this number, as this would help tremendously. She wasn't convinced: 'I'll eat my hat if it works.' Happily, it did work – in fact, dramatically so. Her sleep improved, her pain reduced and she was calmer and less cross. When I asked about the hat, she claimed not to have any edible ones.

We live in a culture where we tend to put lifestyle and health in different boxes. Doctors deal with health and we ourselves live life. This division has occurred because healthcare is taken for granted as being free and able to deal with anything. With chronic pain, however, we discover that medicine has its limits. The new perspective we need to consider is one of putting everything together in one big box.

Sometimes we don't see something because we are so used to it, it becomes invisible to us. Sometimes we don't think there is a choice, and at other times we don't want to see it in the first place. All these things can conspire to create a blind spot in our thinking. It is common to fight against limitation and carry on regardless. As I pointed out in the Introduction, so many people go flat out until they have no choice but to rest. When I point out the damage this is causing, they often say, 'Wow, that's me exactly; I hadn't thought of it like that.' Or they say, 'My partner keeps telling me that, but I don't listen.'

We cannot see much when we are hard up against it. As a demonstration, try holding up a hand about a couple of centimetres in front of your face – this may feel a bit silly but it's worth it. With your hand this near your face, you cannot see much at all: it's so close that you can't see the detail of your hand, and you certainly can't see beyond it. All you can see is what is to the sides. But move the hand further away and you can see it in detail, as well as seeing everything around it. As the saying goes, you can't see the wood for the trees – and I'm sure this demonstration would work standing right in front of a tree as well. We will revisit this idea later when we look at stress and relaxation in Chapters 5 and 6.

When you step back and look at the bigger picture of life, you will hopefully see that there are more factors out there than you have thought of. These will often be issues that only you can address, sometimes with help, but ultimately you are in charge. Perhaps they are non-medical issues that make your condition worse or harder to cope with, such as stress at work or struggling to accept change. Everything is important simply because it affects you, and anything that affects you is relevant to health. As has been said above, health affects life, and life affects health. If you cannot change your health, try changing your life and seeing what happens. A lifestyle change is a part of the health jigsaw that only you can change, and it might be the very change that unsticks you.

Models of chronic pain

There are some important models that can be used to describe the bigger picture that I have been talking about. These are now appearing in textbooks and in PowerPoint presentations at conferences – an important step forward because it means that the medical world is changing and taking on a more holistic approach. This of course does not mean your pain consultant will be wearing a kaftan and doing yoga in front of you, but it does mean that he or she will recognize that life issues are important in dealing with pain. The model that most people working in pain services know is the biopsychosocial model (Figure 1.1). This simply says that life with pain affects people in a number of ways. I like to describe it as a map of life with chronic pain.

'Bio' relates to our bodies and physical or biological aspects. 'Psycho', or psychological, concerns thoughts and feelings, and the 'social' bit is about other people. When I ask people to fill this pain map in, the busiest section is always the psychological sphere. I've found that frustration is the most commonly identified emotional issue. Anger, guilt and not being believed also tend to be added quickly.

My way of describing how this plays out is like this. You feel fine (bio), so you think that you'll do some gardening (psycho). So you garden away (bio) and, after a while, you feel some more pain (bio),

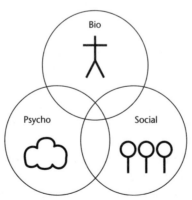

Figure 1.1 The biopsychosocial model (adapted from Engel)

but think, 'I've started so I need to finish' (psycho) and, 'What would the neighbours think? (psychosocial). So you continue gardening and fight against the pain (biopsycho) until you feel awful (bio) and have to give up. You go into the house feeling grumpy (psycho) and then snap at your partner (social). You are in pain and you have a grumpy evening (biopsychosocial). When you feel better again you think, 'I'll just finish that gardening' (psycho). Your partner says, 'Be careful – remember last time' (social), which annoys you (psycho), so you think that you'll show your partner you can do it (psycho) and, guess what, the whole process repeats. The simple act of gardening becomes a really big issue that is riddled with stress and expectation.

And it's not just gardening – everything in life is in fact biopsychosocial. While I am writing this sitting in a chair (bio), I am thinking about what to write and worrying about the deadline (psycho), and also thinking about my cat, who is poorly (social). So it is easy to see that the biopsychosocial model provides an excellent way to describe the bigger picture. If something arises, we need to trace it through all the spheres. Also, a change for the better in one sphere will improve the whole picture.

Some people argue that there should be more spheres, such as environmental or workplace, where stress or money issues might arise. I agree. This is a good model because it looks at the big picture, but it is limited by its three categories. As a result, I have come up with an altogether messier 'knot' model that I am still developing. I know it's messy, but life is like that. I have, however, had feedback that people with pain can relate to it and I also hope this knot model conveys some of the feelings experienced in living with chronic pain.

The big knot

I spent most of my childhood untangling knots. I'm not very good at it, though. In the 1970s, I used to fly double-stringed kites with my dad. These were fantastic, especially compared to the old box kites that just used to sit in the air doing nothing. I could do lots of tricks, dive-bomb my brothers and have a great time. But when the kites crashed, the knots were even more spectacular than the tricks. They took ages to untangle before we could fly again, and this seems to me be a good metaphor for life with chronic pain.

Living with any chronic condition is like a big tangled knot, with many issues wrapped around and entwined with each other (Figure 1.2). It's not tidy. There are the symptoms of the condition, worries about the condition, physical limitations, frustration, worry about what people think, anxiety, sleep issues, much stress, dietary implications, low mood, beliefs relating to the pain, relationship issues, loss of fitness, fear of activity and difficulty accepting change. It also means that you cannot do the equivalent of flying your own kite while the strings are still tangled. This is the big picture of life with pain.

Living with a downturn in health means that you have more on your plate (a bigger knot) than you used to. This, in turn, usually means more stress, and we all know that stress heightens our emotions and makes pain worse. Bear in mind that part of the knot might have been with you for a while. For example, a change in health may be the straw that breaks the camel's back of a difficult relationship.

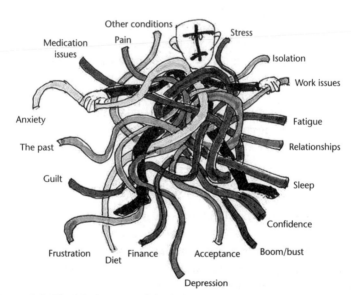

Figure 1.2 The big knot model of chronic pain

The picture can be confused by the fact that pain tends to get all the blame for the situation. This is not to say that the pain isn't a central factor, but often the whole knot gets labelled as 'pain'. The symptoms of your condition are probably the most obvious strands in the knot, and they are the ones you go to the doctor about. But they are not the whole knot, and it is easy to get tied up with the pain strand and lose sight of everything else. Sadly, that's what my tuba player was doing.

Unravelling the knot

This book is about helping you to manage your chronic pain and cope better. In short, this means unravelling your knot, but this can be a tricky business. If you pull hard on one end, the knot often gets tighter. But if you cannot accept the knot, if you pretend that it isn't there, then it will tangle you up even more.

As a child, I wasn't very good at knots because I wanted to find the one simple end that would magically unravel the whole tangle, thereby saving me time. But the lesson I learnt was to follow one strand at a time and work with what I could. Like any healing process, we need to untangle the knot of life gently, bit by bit. Pain is the obvious strand, but it might be that something else needs to be untangled first. Or it might be that we just need to work with whatever end is presenting itself to us right now.

This 'one strand' theme is very important. Don't beat yourself up by trying to fix everything in one go. Instead, try to focus on just one thing at a time that you can understand or do. In all my sessions, I ask people to look for one single thing that they can take away – something that's one strand of their knot. Any more than this, and it gets too hard. Just like knots, a person's situation can seem overwhelming, but focusing on one strand at a time and doing what you can do at this point is a realistic way forward.

This is an extension of the biopsychosocial model of health mentioned above. It reflects the fact that the reality of health is that we have to actually live with it rather than just have the condition in isolation. As pain affects life and life affects pain, we need to start untangling our knots.

Summary

All the factors involved in the knot are directly relevant to pain because pain is produced by the complex interplay of the body, nervous system and mind. How we think and what we believe at an unconscious level makes a tremendous difference to the way the central nervous system processes information. We will explore this more in Chapter 2, on understanding pain.

2

Understanding pain

Nothing in life is to be feared, it is only to be understood. Now is the time to understand more, so that we may fear less.

Marie Curie

Pain is nature's way of saying 'Stop!' It hits us in such an awful way that we have to obey it. That's a good thing because it forces us to prevent further damage and do things to heal ourselves. Think of broken limbs, bruises, burns, sprains, strains and even mysterious new pains – they all force us to pay attention, change what we are doing, seek help and change our behaviour. Pain protects, and we would be dead without it.

In the same way that people complain about the council and bad design, you might exclaim: 'You'd have thought they could have devised a better system by now!' Perhaps a set of warning lights or a buzzer would do the trick. If you were in charge of such things, however, you might point out that people do not obey lights and alarms. When the stakes are high, when survival is the issue, we need something drastic such as pain.

To appreciate the importance of pain, consider the plight of people who have a congenital insensitivity to pain. In this rare condition, people do not feel pain or do not react to it, fantastic though that sounds. They therefore do not know when they have, for example, been burnt or injured, and they do not get a prompt from a new pain that something requires a visit to the doctor. Sadly, many die young from injuries they have not felt or reacted to.

Like stress and fear, pain is one of a family of basic reactions that enable us to survive. I call these the caveman responses. All the caveman responses are obvious when you have them, but how you come to have them is more complicated than you might think. This is important, because the fact that pain is complex in nature means there are opportunities which you probably are not aware of to make improvements. People often tell me 'pain is pain', but when you understand it properly, there's far more to it than that.

Acute and chronic pain

There two sorts of pain: acute and chronic. Both are obviously pain, but it is crucial to understand that they are very different from each other.

'Acute' does not mean sharp and pointy like a triangle; it simply means short term. Acute pain is caused by damage or a change in the body, and as the damage heals, the pain goes away. In many ways, acute pain is what nature intends pain to be used for. It warns of damage and forces us to rest and immobilize the damaged area. There is usually something to 'see', either externally, such as a plaster cast, or internally by using an X-ray or other scan. With acute pain, the pain we feel is usually in proportion to what is happening in the body.

On the whole, acute pain is quite simple, it 'behaves' predictably and goes away with time. A classic saying associated with acute pain is 'the issue is in the tissue'. This means that the main source lies in some physical part of the body. And with acute pain, painkillers tend to be an effective treatment.

Chronic pain is a completely different beast. 'Chronic' does not mean old and creaking like a ship; it simply means long term. Chronic pain can start with an acute injury or be caused by a condition that develops over time. Thousands of conditions are associated with chronic pain; common ones are arthritis, back pain, fibromyalgia and neuropathic pain. Many people, however, have long-term pain that does not fit neatly into a diagnostic box – sometimes the diagnosis is just 'chronic pain'.

As described in the Introduction, 'chronic pain' is an umbrella term that simply relates to how long the pain has lasted. It is impossible to write one description that will fit everyone exactly, but common themes of chronic pain are a nervous system that has gone on to a kind of 'red alert', a pain that does not normally mean new damage (it is important to check that this is the case), pain that increases and decreases, with good days, bad days and flare-ups, a lack of anything to see so that people look well, and scans that reveal little or nothing. Chronic pain is largely related to how the nervous system is processing information from the body. Sadly, in this situation painkillers are poor pain assassins!

The main differences between the two types of pain are summarized in Table 2.1.

Table 2.1 The differences between acute and chronic pain

Acute pain	Chronic pain
Less than 3–6 months	More than 3–6 months
Pain declines with time	Pain level goes up and down
Clear link with the physical	Mainly nervous system
Issue in the tissue	Issue in the nervous system
Analgesics work well	Analgesics are less effective
Visible	Invisible
Hurt = harm	Hurt = may not mean harm to the body, depending on your condition

Unfortunately, like everything in life, this distinction is not all black and white. There are of course situations where people might have recurring acute episodes. This is better described as a long-term underlying condition – a kind of chronic–acute. Often, however, such people might have constant background pain, which I would call chronic pain. Ultimately, it does not really matter because all these pain types benefit from what we look at in this book.

In the book, I have to generalize, but you will be able to pick out the bits that are relevant to you. Part of understanding your own specific condition is to know the status of the pain you feel. As I pointed out above, pain is sometimes just pain and not a reflection of new damage. With many conditions, hurt does not equal harm, but you need to check this out with a professional clinician who knows about your condition. It is also important to remember that pain is a protective alarm, so new pains and different pains need to be taken seriously and checked out professionally.

The sources of pain

Any change in the body can potentially cause pain, but the pain can be classified into four basic categories of how it is being caused. The categories are:

- nociceptive: in which nerves called nociceptors are stimulated by impacts or aggravations in the tissue around them to produce an electrical signal;
- neuropathic: in which the nerves themselves are damaged or affected;
- inflammatory: in which the autoimmune system produces inflammation to protect you against what it mistakenly thinks is a foreign invader, such as a virus;
- central/nociplastic: in which the nervous system becomes more sensitive and produces pain more readily

Each of these is usually associated with different kinds of pain sensation. For example neuropathic pain might be described as shooting or burning.

The source of pain is just the beginning of the pain journey, and what happens after that is up to the nervous system. It is possible to have a cause for pain but not feel it. There is a famous case of a man who had been shot but did not realize until a bullet was found in his chest during surgery decades later for something entirely unconnected. Changes in the body sometimes happen slowly, so the nervous system gets used to them; at other times, small changes are felt as large pains. This can all seem seem very mysterious but many pain puzzles can be explained by the fact that chronic pain has more to do with the way in which the nervous system processes information than what is happening in the body.

What goes up must (sometimes) come down

The central nervous system consists of the brain and the spinal cord. It is a bit like a person's internal computer system. It is vastly powerful. It takes all the information being fed in to it from body parts via the peripheral nervous system, processes this and gives a response that it 'thinks' is appropriate. Put simply, it processes inputs and gives outputs. If you hit your thumb with a hammer, that's an input: the action produces an electrical signal that was generated by hitting the nerve endings in your thumb. The pain felt is the result of that information being relayed to the brain and processed – it's the output of the system.

Throw a ball in the air and you know that *what goes up must come down*. But with pain, the information being sent up to the brain might not in fact get up there; it might get filtered out. This is why some people look like they should be in a lot of pain but aren't. For others, the same message that goes up the nervous system to the brain might come back as light as a feather or as heavy as an anvil – the level of pain felt all depends on what sense the brain makes of it. The new science of pain shows that the nervous system filters information in or out and processes it in different ways. It explains why some people react strongly to inputs and others do not.

Core sensitization

Everything we experience is traffic on the roads of our nervous system, so the picture can be very complicated, and the nervous system can be very difficult to argue with. That's why pain medicine struggles. If you trick the nervous system for a while with analgesics, it may work out what you are doing and change the sensitivity levels so the pain increases again. Pain, stress and emotions are all in the same traffic jam in the nervous system, so it is no surprise that they affect each other.

In chronic pain, the central nervous system may have gone on to red alert – known as core sensitization. This doesn't mean that someone is a 'sensitive flower', it just means that the brain has decided to produce pain in response to 'non-noxious' – non-damaging – stimuli. The result is that things which shouldn't hurt, do.

For example, a person with chronic regional pain syndrome might find that even the brush of clothes against the skin can be painful. A man with this condition in one of my groups could hold his own arm, but when I touched him on the shoulder to say hello he almost jumped through the roof! This highlights that it is not just about the input, but also about what it means to the brain.

A couple of metaphors might help in understanding this better. Chronic pain is like a record player. The record is your body, and like all bodies it has 'scratches' on it. The stylus represents the nerves that pick up what is happening in the body and send an electrical signal to the amplifier, which is the central nervous system. The record player will then play the sound – the pain – out through the speaker. In chronic pain, the volume control is turned up high so that any scratch on the record creates a huge crackle or screech. The volume can be turned up just because we are, perhaps, more stressed; if we are calmer, the volume turns down. If we overdo it, this puts a longer temporary scratch on the record, and if we think about pain all day, the sound gets louder and louder.

Or if you are a computer fan, you could think of typing an X on your computer and getting XXXXXXXXXX back on your screen. But pain can be a strange thing, and people with neuropathic pain sometimes put an X in and get XYZABC back. The important point to grasp is that what you are feeling is an output from a system rather than a reflection of what is actually happening in your body; it's just a feeling. This is important because hurt does not always mean harm; your physiotherapist, for example, may tell you this from time to time.

Threat sum

There is a lot of complexity in theories about pain, but it all seems to boil down to how the brain is assessing the threat of damage. The official medical definition of pain says that it's about 'actual or potential tissue damage', which means that the brain is assessing current damage or expecting damage to occur.

I like to view this as the brain doing a quick bit of maths, adding up all the threats and then giving a response based on the total. However, not everything is a threat; in fact, most inputs are not relevant to assessing potential damage to the body, which is what pain is supposed to be for. Many of the items in the threat sum might be based on events in the past – it's just that the brain remembers them and includes them in its calculations.

Powerful as it is, the brain can be a bit off-target at times, hanging on to old ideas and patterns just in case. This is also why trauma is such a big issue with chronic pain. A person who has been traumatized at any stage in their life may have unwittingly been on red alert for years on end. If this is you, one-to-one professional help is important to help unravel this – when you are ready.

Primary and secondary suffering – the 'three thumbs'

One of the focuses in helping people with pain is getting past the idea that pain is a fixed thing that they are stuck with. I'm often told, 'Yes, but pain is pain', which makes it sound as if nothing about it can be changed. 'Pain is pain' reflects a view of pain as the inevitable consequence of a medical condition, and many people think that only doctors can help with a 'medical' thing like pain.

The trouble is that we define issues by the tools we have to deal with them. Medicine has always been seen as the 'tool' to deal with pain, so when it stops helping, it's easy to give up and see pain as a failure of medicine, and believe that mere mortals like us cannot possibly do anything about it. 'Pain is pain' keeps people trapped in feeling helpless, and this view doesn't get us anywhere.

Pain is a complex experience that affects people, and not just bits of bodies. It is an experience, not a physical thing. People's experience of pain has two basic aspects: sensory and emotional. Pain practitioners refer to this as *primary* and *secondary* suffering. This means that when you hit your thumb with a hammer, there is the throb (sensory response – the primary part) and then possibly some bad language (emotional response – the secondary part).

The emotional aspect of pain is an important and helpful response. Imagine breaking your leg while larking around trying to jump over a wall. It hurts of course, but it's also frightening, and this is a good thing because it can force you to be more careful in future – and use the gate instead. The fear after the damage has occurred is useful because it stops you from doing that sort of thing again.

With pain, if the emotional response is different, then the pain is different. To illustrate this, think about three different hammer and thumb situations.

1 You hit yourself with your hammer – your thumb throbs and you swear out loud.
2 A stranger sneaks into your shed, grabs the hammer and hits your thumb – you throb and swear, but you also feel angry and shocked.
3 Your four-year-old son is 'helping' you but misses his target and hits your thumb instead – your thumb is throbbing just the same, but you reassure your son that everything is OK.

So the same sensory 'input' has very different emotions attached depending on the context. We could even go as far as saying that the pain was different each time, or maybe that there was a different experience each time. I am sure we would all find that the pain was worst in the second case. So pain is not just what you feel, but how you react at that time, and that is based on what the situation means.

This distinction between primary and secondary suffering is crucial to improving pain. The key idea here is that the sensory input is always modified by the context, and we need to make a distinction between the pain and the effect it causes. For example, a soldier who gets shot might scream out in pain but then smile a bit when he realizes that it means he will get shipped home; or the farmer who loses a finger in a machine may not feel the pain until he is safe in the hospital getting his finger sewn back on.

In pain management, although we can work towards dealing with the physical side of the pain, we also need to improve our reactions to it – so we tackle the total experience of pain (the 'ouch' and our reaction to it). This way of looking at pain also implies that an improved reaction will actually start to modify and even block the pain signal.

A lorry load of pain

We have seen how emotion is an integral part of the pain experience, and indeed, as we saw in the Introduction, the medical definition of pain is that it is an unpleasant sensory and emotional experience. This is extremely important because what pain means, especially in terms of its threat value, has everything to do with the pain we feel. The pain cannot be split from the experience of the pain.

But with chronic pain the emotional response can grow enormously with time. The sensation of pain is potentially accompanied by an avalanche of: not again; I hate this; it might never go away; I'm desperate for it to improve; I'm trying not to feel it; why me?; everyone judges me; this isn't me; nothing works; maybe I'm mad; maybe I'm bad. The constant conjunction of sensation and reaction means that the total experience of pain is like being hit with a brick every time. The physical hurt and the emotional hurt become rolled up into one experience that we call pain. The build-up of pain and the reaction to it can become a powerful reflex that we experience without being able to separate it into its parts.

The emotional response can also rumble on without the sensation being present. Some people get so used to being in pain that they assume they are even when they are not. In such situations, medical scans and pain diaries can be helpful to establish what is really going on.

The build-up of sensation and reaction, and everything that feeds in to the overall picture, is like a lorry. The engine unit is the sensation, and the trailers rumble behind containing reactions to pain, thoughts and feelings about life, and situations that are stressful.

Pain science

Current pain science has overturned the old thinking that pain was something that a person was a passive victim of. There are two strands to current thoughts: the gate theory, and the neuromatrix.

Gate theory concerns how the signal for pain ascends to the brain but is, on its journey, modified by having to pass through 'gates' that are opened or closed by instructions coming down from the brain. Put far too simply, this says that we will have less pain when we are happy. It also explains how when a mother is rubbing her child's arm, a signal is created that closes a pain gate and interrupts the pain signalling – an idea that helps to explain how TENS (transcutaneous electrical nerve stimulation) machines work.

The idea behind the neuromatrix is that 'pain' relates to a matrix of different parts of the brain that 'light up' when the brain thinks they are needed. The brain matrix that we call pain is like a band playing a tune. It learns the tune over time and requires less and less instruction from the conductor before it starts to play. This is an idea I've borrowed from the excellent book *Explain Pain* (Butler and Moseley, 2013). Here, then, pain is all to do with how the brain interprets the information it gets. The key to this approach is understanding threat – the original suggestion was that if the brain understands how the pain happens, this will reduce its threat value and thereby set the band off less often. And even when the band is playing, the person will realize that this is just a brain event called pain, rather than a physical thing in the body.

So, to recap, pain is not something concrete in the body, but a response from the brain based largely on an assessment of what it thinks is happening and what needs to happen to protect you. In acute pain, the brain tends to get this right, but with chronic pain there is a highly variable relationship between what is happening in the body and what you feel – in short, the brain can get it wrong. One man once described this to me as 'a false red alert'.

We have also identified pain as an experience consisting of sensory and emotional components: it's not just the 'ouch', but everything in the trailers attached to the pain lorry. And this affects how pain is felt because our mood affects what the brain wants to know and how the nervous system sends information to it. Removing or improving some of the trailer contents may simplify the message and improve the pain.

The PC Tom matrix – an illustration of the science of pain

To summarize the science of pain in a way that I would understand it, let me introduce you to a typical British town centre with a CCTV camera trained on the area outside the local pub. In the local police station, a semi-retired police officer called Tom is watching his screens to monitor what is happening outside the pub (Figure 2.1). If there is any kind of trouble, he presses an alarm that sends the police to that location. When the police go, they usually close the pub and may even arrest the suspects, or ban them from the pub for a while. Related to the science of pain, Tom is the brain/central nervous system, the camera is the peripheral nervous system and the area outside the pub is the body.

Like all central nervous systems, Tom wants to keep his town safe. How he interprets what he sees depends on many issues. As he has been around for a while, he knows the town; he knows certain of its characters and has probably arrested a few of them in his time. Like all police and all brains, Tom has learnt to expect certain things, spot patterns and predict what he thinks will happen. And this is all good – to a point.

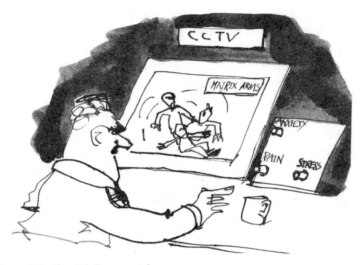

Figure 2.1 The PC Tom matrix

Sometimes Tom will see a fight and rightly press the alarm button. Other times, he might think there is bound to be a fight – because there always is on a Saturday night – so he presses the alarm as soon as he sees a few folk gathering. And sometimes Tom gets stressed and tired – as lots of people with chronic pain do. He then tends to get a bit twitchy and presses the alarm button as soon as anything happens. In addition, if there is a fight outside this pub, Tom might look at his other screens and assume that there will be fights outside the other pubs in the town, so he presses the alarm button to send the police teams to all those places as well. If he is having an especially bad time, he might start zooming in on smaller details, such as buskers, looking for trouble to break out. And in an extreme situation when he is really wound up, a busker with a guitar case might look like someone with a gun, so Tom will hurriedly press the alarm.

At a particularly bad point, Tom got sent to the doctor and was given medicine to calm him down. Unfortunately, this had side effects that meant he felt dreadful. Sometimes it also meant he was too dopey to see a fight properly or would press the alarm really early, thinking there was still likely to be a fight even though he could not really see any sign of one.

But what if we could make Tom happy and relaxed? He might not watch the cameras so keenly and respond to the slightest detail. If he puts on his recording of Abba played on the pan pipes – and there is such a thing – he might sit back, relax and lose himself in the haunting melodies. Or maybe he is an Elvis fan, or he chooses to bring his stamp collection in to look at during quiet moments. Whatever he does, he will be distracted and not notice so much of what's happening and overreact to it. Then his partner might pop in and give him a soothing neck massage; when this happens he doesn't bother looking at the screens as closely (like interrupting the pain signal in the gate theory).

Tom could also be sent on a course to learn that, from a socio-logical perspective, sending the police in to sort out fights may only make the situation worse – like education on pain explaining to people how reacting to it differently will benefit them. So when Tom sees a little fight, he might just think that it will actually finish soon. Even with a big fight, Tom might think that this always happens on a Saturday night and sending the police in won't make much difference – the people fighting won't hurt anyone else, and the police are only going to make it worse if they wade in. So Tom chooses to let things be and enjoy the evening instead.

Is it real?

All this talk of signals and processing and PC Tom's matrix and setting off alarms is one thing, but people still get hung up on whether pain is real. It is easy to feel like a fraud when there is nothing to see, but be reassured that the nature of chronic pain, unlike acute pain where there is current damage, is mostly to do with the way the nervous system is working. People expect to see something to account for their pain because that has been their previous experience of pain. Despite all the pain science, the idea of pain as an output from the brain is still unfamiliar to them.

There is a joke about a pain consultant who goes to see an ortho-paedic surgeon complaining of a long-term painful knee. When asked where exactly the pain is, the pain consultant points to his head. They both know what he means – the knee is where the problem started, but it's the brain that is making him feel it.

Phantom limb pain – when someone feels pain in a part of their body that they have lost – is another way of showing that the pain is being constructed by the brain. When information on an irritation in the stump reaches the brain, the brain often matches it up to its internal map and gives its owner pain in a foot they no longer have. One client said that massaging the missing limb helped them. Another said a bag of frozen peas on the missing foot helped – bizarre, but it all illustrates how pain is ultimately produced by the brain.

The idea that body events are more real than brain events is a cultural construction that is slowly changing. The reality is that pain is whatever you feel, regardless of how it is being caused. If you feel it, it's real. Whether or not a cause can be found is another matter entirely.

Summary

Pain is not just pain. It is a complex experience that affects people and not just bits of bodies. Anything that affects you affects pain, and anything that affects pain affects you. Whatever pain is or is not, it is the experience of living with it that counts. Anything we can do to improve life will improve pain in one way or another.

Part 2
MANAGING

3

Booby traps

I guess man is the only kind of varmint sets his own trap, baits it, then steps in it.

John Steinbeck

The following chapters deal with the major booby traps of chronic pain and what to do about them. By 'booby trap' I mean something that catches us out when we are just trying to get on with our normal lives (Figure 3.1). A basic feature of every booby trap in pain management is that it creates an unpleasant cycle (a vicious cycle) that feeds on itself and gets worse with time.

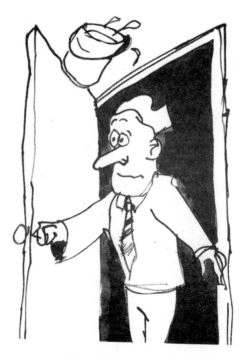

Figure 3.1 A classic booby trap

The big three booby traps are boom–bust, stress and lack of sleep. These three are the big ones that lie in wait for us and really catch us out. When they do, they often lead to other issues by dragging fitness, mood and everything and anything else down with them.

They affect how our pain is managed too as they are unlikely to be considered in a standard medical setting, especially as there is rarely enough time to deal with them. Issues such as stress and lack of sleep are often seen as just inevitable side issues. However, they are central to the whole situation of pain. And if you do something about them, the whole picture of your pain will change for the better. There is a simple argument here: if we can't change pain by directly 'attacking' it, such as with medicines – and this is likely to be the case – then we need to go round to the back door and do what else we can, rather than rely on medicines alone. In a world dominated by 'painkillers', it's easy to think that these 'back door' approaches are second best, but I believe that they are 'first best'. The ones I am going to describe have no side effects and no costs – they just involve a different way of thinking and a little effort.

4

Pacing

Slow but steady wins the race.

Aesop

Pacing is a huge topic, so I've split this big chapter into manageable chunks. In fact, I've paced myself!

The boom–bust cycle

A change in health often means that we cannot do as much as we used to, but it doesn't stop us trying!

It's a bit like driving. Imagine that your car has been fitted with a limiter so that you can no longer go at the national speed limit like everyone else. It's hard to plod along at, say, 40 m.p.h. when you know your car can go much faster, at least for a bit before the limiter cuts in. And imagine that when it does cut in, it might cut out and leave you stuck at the side of the road for a day or so. It's tough when everyone else is whizzing by. You'll be frustrated because you also used to zip past the plodders. You may feel under pressure to do more and go faster. The people behind may be flashing their lights to try to speed you up, although the irony here is that we are usually sensitive about our own speed, so we really want to flash ourselves to go faster.

No one wants to be limited, so it is natural to fight against it. In this battle, we try to do everything we used to, often more. Things get worse, pain keeps winning, but many of us just keep fighting on. In the car analogy, you drive flat out all the time so the speed limiter cuts in more and more. In time your top speed drops to 30 and you spend longer stranded at the roadside.

This is the boom–bust pattern. It's amazing how common it is. The classic story is that on a good day people do as much as they can until the pain stops them, and then they are forced to rest until they recover sufficiently. And then they're off again, pushing to the limit and inevitably crashing out once more. It's like waking up and running into a wall.

In pain management, the 'boom–bust' cycle is officially known as the overactivity–rest cycle, but there is more to it than just a physical aspect. A lot of stress and emotion is involved too. This can floor us because it means that we never switch off. Even when we are forced to rest the body, the mind is still whirring away like a revving engine that stirs up distress. This wears us out at every level: physically, mentally, emotionally.

Most people say that their overriding emotion is frustration. Others talk about anger, guilt or just trying to ignore what has happened. Whatever the emotion, it often overrides the competing need to manage pain. If this pattern were sold as a trendy T-shirt slogan, it might read:

Frustration
Pain
Collapse
Repeat

You might think of your own version, but the key is that this is a repeating pattern. Figure 4.1 is what this looks like in graph form.

From this graph, you can see that cycling between boom and bust can cause a gradual reduction in function and increase in

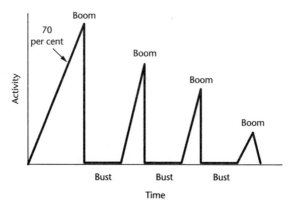

Figure 4.1 The boom–bust cycle

pain. The booms gradually get shorter, and the busts eventually last longer. This is a miserable experience that causes even more frustration, anxiety and stress. Ironically, the worse it gets, the harder people fight to stay the same. This is understandable but it leads to a downward spiral in which pain gets worse with time.

Booming and busting is not a disease, it's not boombustitis; rather, it's a personal reaction to limitation. That reaction is entirely natural and based on the moral principles of 'decent' folk – that we should fight against challenges, try our best and maintain standards. But this can be counterproductive, especially when we are 'heated up' by stress and worry. In uncertain times, it is natural to want certainty – this is partly why people doggedly follow tenets such as 'finish what you start'. We'll look at this again later, but for now it is important to know that we can bully ourselves with old rules such as 'standards have to be maintained' and follow them too rigidly regardless of how they affect us.

Why it gets worse

There are several possible reasons why the picture gets worse with time. Specific clinical reasons for this need, of course, to be checked with your doctor, but over and above these there are a number of important issues to understand. Contrary to popular opinion, you *can* do something about these. The elephant in the room is that we simply get worn out. The mental, physical and emotional strain of living flat out all the time wears us down, and we lose our ability to bounce back as our internal resources diminish.

Living flat out, even when it looks like you are resting, means that a cycle becomes established. Stress, lack of sleep, loss of fitness and difficult emotions all chase each other around. With time, the battle to stay the same gets increasingly desperate, which revs everything up. So it's not a surprise that things get worse with time. Regardless of pre-existing health conditions, anyone who is stressed, does not sleep much, loses fitness and feels anxious will start to show it physically. A friend told me that when she was training to be a doctor in the mad old days when 90-hour training weeks were a norm, a number of her fellow students started to experience pain and fatigue.

People simply get worn out. This is important because it is easy to confuse the effect of boom–bust with a worsening condition. Again, it is important to check this with your doctor to be sure about your own condition, and to reassure you so that you feel less fearful and less stressed. But the good news is that it will help if you tame the boom–bust cycle because it is not a disease in itself; and you can do this. Although for a bit of fun you could start telling people you've got yet another diagnosis – boombustitis!

Neuroplastic change

The big new idea to introduce here is *neuroplastic change*. This concept is a relatively new development in pain science. It means that the nervous system (the 'neuro' bit) learns and then adapts (the 'plastic' bit). We need this because the nervous system learns beneficial things through practice, like how to catch a ball or how to drive. It can also help with potentially painful things; think, for instance, about how school dinner ladies seem to have asbestos hands. But like plastic, the system can bend one way or another, and this is when we need to outwit it to avoid problems.

To understand this, think of the pain system as a kindly parent who wants to protect you. Imagine your little loved one doing something they shouldn't: you gently tell them not to, but they still do it, and then you tell them off again. Next time they are heading for the knife drawer, you will say something sooner, and if they continue to do it, you will tell them off sooner and sooner until the stage where you spring into action as soon as you see that glint of mischief in their eyes. Pain is the same. It's trying to protect you. If you ignore it, it protects you more quickly and more loudly. The way to change this is to teach it that you do things differently. In this context, doing things differently means teaching your nervous system that you do not have to wait to be told off! This is where pacing comes in.

It is also about breaking the conditioned reflex. If you do too much every time you go for a walk, your brain will spot a pattern and give you pain when it calculates you are off walking again.

Another way of referring to this change is as core sensiti-zation. This does not mean you're a sensitive flower; rather, it's about how the central (core) nervous system learns to react more quickly and strongly to inputs from the world. In some cases, such as chronic regional pain syndrome, it can mean someone has a very sensitive part of their body so that even a light touch hurts. For others, the system may be generally sensitive to every-thing, and this is particularly so in fibromyalgia and related conditions.

Living at the limit of your capabilities means that your limit declines over time. This is often considered to be part of a condition and therefore something that we cannot affect. But generally speaking, it is not part of a condition, and you *can* do something about it.

So now let's look at the 'P' word – pacing.

What pacing is

The boom–bust cycle happens when we try too hard to beat pain and be in control; pacing is a way to tame the cycle and regain proper control. It involves adapting to change, mostly by stopping what you are doing before the pain stops you. But as everyone tells me, this is easy to say, but hard to do.

Pacing is a real 'Marmite' topic. People love it or hate it. Most hate it to start with, and some continue to do so, possibly because they have encountered a self-management zealot or are afraid that pacing amounts to giving in. Others say they cannot do it because they have no choice to alter the patterns in their life. These strong reactions against the simple idea of taking things a bit easier shows just how it prods a sensitive button.

I have met a few people who hate even the word 'pacing', a bit like the Knights who say Nii in the film *Monty Python and the Holy Grail* hate the word 'it' – 'it' literally scares them off. One lady I worked with just couldn't abide the word, and our session ground to a halt until we decided to rename it 'choicing'. She was much happier with that and then used the approach to change her life. Another person said to me in all seriousness, 'It's a swear word.' The moral of the story is to call it what you want to.

The big issue with pacing is that we have to deal with change. No one likes change, and that might explain why the technique can be unpopular. But if nothing changes, then nothing changes. As the ancient Chinese philosopher Lao Tzu once said: 'If you do not change direction, you may end up where you are heading.' If you are starting to worry that this will change (there's that word again) your life in strange ways, remember that the real aim is not to avoid situations that may cause pain, and therefore cut things out of your life, but to put you in control by maximizing your choices. It's about making the best of a life that has been limited by pain. So it's up to you what you do with these ideas – it's your choice.

Pacing should, however, be a familiar idea. We talk about running a race at the right pace, or overpacing when we do too much too soon. The most famous example is Aesop's fable about the Hare and the Tortoise who run a race. The Hare keeps sprinting and then resting, while the Tortoise just plods along and eventually wins, the lesson being that 'slow and steady wins the race'. But none of us wants to plod along, especially when many people seem to be Hares. Indeed, most people I work with are Hares.

I would like to introduce a third animal here – the cunning Fox. Just like youngsters running cross-country races at school, he finds sneaky ways around situations. If he were in the race he would take a taxi, get someone else to run a bit for him, take a short cut or even change the rules or ask the question, 'Why is winning so important anyway?' I would like to suggest that we forget the frantic Hares and plodding Tortoises and all become a bit more Foxy instead.

In practice, as I said above, the great big basic idea of pacing is to work within your limits so that you stop before the pain stops you. Not to avoid pain but to adapt by making choices based on your values. Being more in control reflects the fact that your needs are important to you and that you will be kinder to yourself. Rather than plodding, the aim is to do more in the end because there will be fewer bad days. It is also about doing more of what you want to do and less of what you feel obliged to do.

My version of pacing is simply to work to 70 per cent of capacity. Obviously, that is impossible to gauge exactly, but it acts as a reminder to stop while there is still fuel in the tank. It is of course up to you what percentage you use, but suffice it to say that 99 per cent will lead to trouble and 10 per cent means you will get virtually nothing done. The '70 per cent' value works well though to make sure that you still have something left in the tank.

The graph in Figure 4.1 showed that the difficulties arise not from doing things per se, but from doing that last little bit extra. Plan things so that you finish before the pain takes over. I know this is not always possible – you can't suddenly stop driving to your destination, for example – but often you will know roughly where your limit is and can plan to it. Unfortunately, we often either forget to notice our limit, or don't want to notice it. We hope and gamble that somehow it will all be fine.

How to pace

A few relatively simple things can be done to apply the 70 per cent rule and reduce the load on your system. The real battle, however, is overcoming the reluctance to actually apply the big idea and adapt to change. If you have a 'pacing mindset' or have practised pacing, you will do these things naturally without thinking. But if you are not there yet, it is worth outlining them because they might have never occurred to you – especially if you are one of those 100 per cent-non-stop-multitasking-perfectionist-hare-type people. If your brain is not yet in gear, try these ideas out, even a little, and see what happens.

Redefine what counts as a job

Most people will try to finish what they start and do things like they always have done them, but this is doomed to failure. The idea is to break tasks into realistic 'chunks' that you can actually achieve, and then stop when you have done them. Obviously, some things, like crossing the road, are not divisible, but most are if you are prepared to challenge the idea of having to do things the way you have always done them.

Anne tried to clean her whole house every week from top to bottom in a day. She was a self-confessed perfectionist, so cleaning the house was a big undertaking. Not surprisingly, it kept beating her. We looked at a way in which she could keep her standards intact and survive the day. It took a bit of adjusting, but in the end she decided to do one room well each day. She said that she could look at that room and feel she had achieved something. Ironically, when she did a lot more in the house but had to give up before she finished, she felt she had failed because she had not delivered on her rule to 'finish what I start'.

Do a good job

This may sound a bit odd here, but if you think about it, a job is not just the task itself. I was always taught to make sure I looked after the tools I had. And your most useful tool is yourself. Obviously, you don't need to oil yourself and hang yourself up in the garage, but you do need to look after yourself. Imagine an employer expecting his staff to work flat out with no regard for their health – he would soon have no staff.

Beware of saying, 'I'll stop when I finish'; this is a classic lie that people tell themselves, especially under the tyranny of housework that never finishes. Remember that housework *can* finish if you define it as separate tasks rather than an ongoing battle.

Prioritize

This is simply asking, 'What is really important?' Some people think everything is important, but with reduced capacity something has to give. Identifying what needs to be done rather than what you think you ought to do is really important.

I worked with a lady who used to be in the Royal Navy. This is relevant because apparently they clean everything regardless – although so do the army and even some people who are not in the forces. She had a punishing routine, part of which involved damp-dusting all the skirting boards in her large Victorian house. She dreaded doing it but felt she had to. Even her husband did not want her to do it because it left her in a heap.

When we looked at it, she realized that the skirting boards were never that dusty, she was no longer on HMS Housework, and it was one job she could drop. It was a want rather than a need, and in fact the more she thought about it, the more the want faded too. Just dropping one job for now is important because it gets you into the habit of change and realizing that you are allowed to change the rules that enslave you. More on rule-rebellion later!

Run a cost–benefit analysis

This sounds fancy but it's just like shopping in that it's making a decision about whether what you are doing is worth the price you will pay for doing it. Again, it is not about avoiding pain but about making sure that you are tying yourself in with your needs, values and priorities. All you need to do is start asking yourself, 'Is this worth it?' And funnily enough, asking yourself that question is always worth it.

Try switching

Doing the same action repeatedly, or even not moving much at all, is not helpful. It is important to switch between activities so that you use different muscle groups. A good example is swapping between bending and stretching tasks.

Take breaks

Taking a break seems blindingly obvious, but it is easy to get carried away and forget to stop. Breaks literally break up jobs into manageable chunks and give you the mental space to step back and ask yourself some sensible questions such as, 'Why am I doing this? Is it worth it? Could I do it differently? Why don't I have more breaks?'

Working on a computer and doing the housework are special hazards for getting carried away. A neat and simple idea is to set an alarm to remind you to stop.

Make adjustments

People sometimes fixate on doing things in only one way, but a simple practical change can make a huge difference. Simple things like ironing sitting down, batch-cooking so that you freeze meals for later, having a taller chair, a shorter chair, a raised keyboard ... these all make small differences that add up. You will be able to work out which changes to make for yourself.

Knowing when you're at 70 per cent to monitor yourself

Most people say they don't know when to stop, but as I said above – which is worth repeating – this is often because they do not really want to know.

There are two ways of knowing that you are getting near your limit. The first is that you feel things building up, like an increase in pain or a change in mood, which is useful if you feel things before it is too late. However, many people say that there is a delay and that the pain hits them when it is too late, the next day for example. If you are in that category, you will need to work out how much you can usually do before it is too much. If you think, while being active, that you are getting away with something, then you probably aren't. Ideally, you will be able to identify a 'buffer zone' where you know to look out for signs of overdoing it, and also know before you start where your limits usually are.

Unfortunately, some people genuinely do not know where their limits are or exactly what causes them difficulty. In this case, friends or family may be able to tell them. Alternatively, they can keep a 'pain diary'. This is not as miserable as it sounds – it is simply recording what you do and how you feel so that you can look back and see patterns. The more information you put in, the better. You can log activity type and amount, weather, medicine, sleep, food, mood, stress. I suggested this to one group but they all found it too depressing – they missed the point though; this is not to think about the pain, but to find out the pattern and deal with it.

This is a bit of an inexact science, and we will all get it wrong from time to time. Hopefully, you will have some success, and with time you will get it right more often.

Ask for help

Many people think that they are the only person who can do a particular job. Some of this might be about pride, or independence, or not wanting to ask, or maybe it's just habit, but whatever it is, it usually means you will end up doing too much. Sometimes we do need help. And help is often what people want to give. They want to feel useful and hate to see you in difficulty, so they are often desperate to lend a hand. But remember that you may need to compromise and not waste more energy following your helper around to check they are doing it 'properly'.

Knowing when it ends

If you know when something will finish, you can pace yourself to match. Imagine a race where the organizers kept extending the finishing point. That's effectively what a lot of people do to themselves. The finishing point gets extended with 'just a bit more' until you end up exhausted. So it is important to set the task and have the discipline to stop when it is finished. This is the big idea behind baselines, which I will explain very shortly.

Pacing is much maligned because it is associated with ideas of having to slow down and become a Tortoise. I prefer to think of this as adapting. To do this, we need to challenge our rules and change our relationship both with pain and with ourselves.

Baselines . . . goal-setting for mortals

The boom–bust habit shows how we often do what we can until we can't. Baselines set things up so that you can do things until you still can. The idea is that if you keep doing what you can rather than what you cannot, you will benefit from the happy spiral of success feeding success.

Baselines revolve around a simple idea: knowing when something will end means that you can plan to match it and pace yourself. It's the opposite of what shopping with my wife is like! Baselines are a form of goal-setting for pain management, but don't let the terminology put you off. In my experience, baselines are remarkably effective because they can be used to limit pain, to improve how much you do or just to cope better. And who wouldn't want that?

The underlying idea is to radically change your relationship with pain. Rather than using pain as your policeman, you replace 'him' with a realistic distance/time/amount of what you will do. By 'realistic', I mean that the amount you set as your goal needs to be something that you can actually do and repeat. The goal in a baseline is not a dream of what you want to get up to, it is what you can reliably do *right now*. If you change the goal to something that you know you can do with confidence, fear drops out of the equation. This might be fear of failure or fear of pain, or just plain fear, but whatever it is, fear is a primal drive and it is vitally important to reduce it in any way you can.

The change in relationship will allow you to stop monitoring pain all the time and to focus on what you are doing. This is helpful because constantly monitoring pain means that you are always noticing it. Imagine an annoying ticking clock – if you kept checking whether you could still hear it or whether it was getting louder, it would become deafening. Pain is the same.

I believe that baselines work because they tap into our basic natural need to focus on what we are undertaking. If the task is realistic enough, the focus will be on doing that rather than on pain. As an example, I worked with Tom, who kept walking until he could not walk any further. Then, to his embarrassment, his wife had to come and rescue him. His motivation was good – he wanted to get fit again – but the way he was doing it was unwittingly setting him up to fail. He was walking as far as he could until he couldn't – he was effectively setting his goal as the point of maximum pain. As time went by, a boom–bust cycle set in and he gradually got worse.

How to sit in a chair and other tasks

Think of a daily activity you want to improve. It could be walking, doing the housework, sitting, standing, you name it. As an example, let's take sitting in a chair. How long can you sit before things get too sore? It will vary from chair to chair and day to day, but think of a typical length of time. For people who are in doubt, I always suggest 20 minutes, which seems to be the 'golden' time.

Whenever you sit down, look at your watch and then stand up after 20 minutes regardless of whether or not you are in pain. If your initial time proves to be too long, reduce it and stick to that as much as you can – obviously, there will be times when you are not in a position to get up – if you are at the cinema, for example.

With time, your confidence should rise, and you will be able to increase the time by a little bit, say by five minutes. This sounds a tedious process and it takes discipline, but, by focusing on the task of standing up, it takes the focus away from the pain, stops you squirming uncomfortably in your chair and gives you permission to act before the pain gets so bad you have no choice. It also retrains your brain, your nervous system and indeed you into knowing that sitting does not inevitably equate to pain.

Geoff did this with standing. He had neuropathic pain and said that every time he stood up it was unbearable. By deciding on 20 minutes as his baseline, he had something to focus on beyond pain. He also knew how long he would be on his feet for so he could plan ahead and cope better, and it also gave him a unit of 'doing-time' to plan around. Geoff applied this and finally built a greenhouse in his garden that had lain in pieces for years. He brought in tomato plants to give to everyone and was delighted that he had got an important part of his life back.

Above, I mentioned Tom who walked until he couldn't. He decided that his baseline needed to be to a nearby lamp-post and back five times a day, and he stuck to this. We agreed that on a good day he would not go any further, on a slightly bad day he would push himself a little, and on a really bad day he would not even try. This combination meant that he slowly became more confident, rebuilt his fitness and gradually found that his nervous system came off red alert. Tom increased his walking distance in increments, one lamp-post at a time. The last time I saw him, he grinned and told me he had just walked ten miles. This is an exceptionally good news story, but what Tom did and the reasons it worked can apply to everyone to some degree.

I'm always looking to discover what makes people tick because that provides a realistic way of moving forward. Sarah was a good swimmer, but when pain meant she could not do her usual big swim, she gave up completely. We spoke about the importance of swimming in Sarah's life. It was indeed so important that she was quite depressed that she had given up. The 'mountain' that we needed to climb together was to get her back in the pool doing anything, no matter how little. Finally my persistence paid off, and she reluctantly agreed that it was better to do something rather than nothing.

Sarah, like so many people, had an all-or-nothing mindset, and it took a while for the thought 'something is better than nothing' to sink in. Sarah's initial baseline was just to walk in the pool and try a few strokes. Her next baseline was to swim widths, and then lengths. Had Sarah tried to match her old standards straight away, it could all have gone wrong, but at every visit having a baseline meant she knew she would always succeed. Happily, she built up from widths to lengths to fractions of miles. In fact, in the end she reached and then even exceeded her old standard.

The builder in one of my groups was Joe (not Bob), and used to run at jobs and keep going until they were finished. However, he was usually finished too and often had to take the next day off. Joe found that setting a baseline of 30 minutes for whatever he was doing – shovelling, shifting, lifting – meant that he broke up his day into chunks that he and his body could survive. This was vital because, as he relied on physical ability for his livelihood, he needed to make sure he was fit enough to stay in his job.

Neil, a retired decorator in Falkirk, wanted to help his disabled brother by decorating his house, but every time he tried do so, it beat him. He was so desperate to help that it blinded him to the fact that he could do things differently and work in half-hour chunks. He realized that doing the job was more important than how he did it: he didn't have to do it all in one go, as he'd been trying to. Neil was thrilled to tell me that he had managed to finally decorate his brother's house by using his half-hour baseline.

Sam, or as he became known 'Sam Sam the pacing man', ran a small farm in the wilds of North Wales. He kept working and pushing on, fighting his pain, until he collapsed. He then adopted a 20-minute baseline for working, followed by a break. By doing this, he stopped collapsing and, to his doctor's delight, came off 30 painkillers a day – a fantastic result from such a simple change.

The key to baselines is to be consistently realistic so that you learn to expect to succeed in what you are doing. It does not matter how small the baseline is. Tiny is great if it means you keep doing it. Doing a smaller amount more often is much better than doing a lot seldom. Hopefully, though, that will allow you to move on to do more, more often. The main idea is to change the relationship with pain so that it is no longer in charge – you are.

Hopefully, you can see that adopting this simple idea and sticking with it is a way to get back an important part of your life. It is not just about being able to do more, which is great in itself, but also about how doing something that is important to you can help you regain a sense of purpose and a feeling that things can move forward.

Yes, but . . . dealing with objections

Douglas Adams, the genius writer of *The Hitchhiker's Guide to the Galaxy*, said that 'bad news' should power space ships because it travels faster than anything else. I would like to add that 'yes, but' is an equally powerful force that could be used to stop things moving entirely.

Ultimately, pacing – or whatever you want to call it – is simple: it is adapting to change. However, when I bring the subject up, I get things thrown at me, not cabbages or eggs of course; rather, I get pelted with 'yes, but'. Or someone crosses their arms with hostility and tells me in no uncertain terms, 'Yes, but . . . that's easy to say but hard to do.' I reply with my own 'yes, but': 'Yes, but just because it's hard, doesn't mean you can't do it.'

I will briefly list a few of the classic 'yes, buts' and try to throw something sensible back at them. This will not create a miracle change, as change takes time, but it is good to make a start and sow the seeds of rebellion. Remember the Fox – maybe it's time to start to break the rules and think outside the box, or at least glimpse how things could be different.

The irony in all this pacing lark is that we often tell others to 'take it easy' when we do not do it ourselves. This is a good question to dwell on: why don't you do all the good things you tell others to do?

Lack of choice

People often say, 'Yes, but I've got no choice.' There may be very good, practical reasons for this, but there is always something somewhere in a person's life that could be changed for the better. Often 'no choice' is a reflex to fend off those who like to challenge the difficult situation that people have got stuck in. It is a way to avoid the boat getting rocked, but sometimes the boat needs to be rocked. Something has to change otherwise nothing changes – it's up to you. Ironically, there is a choice, and it's yours.

Comfortably uncomfortable

It is easy to get comfortably uncomfortable and not try to make any changes. This is a close cousin of 'no choice'. It is based on the myth of 'better the devil you know than the devil you don't'. Just because something is familiar it is not necessarily better, you're just used to it. In this situation, fear of the unknown prevents progress, but the unknown might be much better than the known. A good start might be to dare to leave something not done, or to do it differently, and see what it feels like. The world will undoubtedly not come to an end, and it might even be a more comfortable situation.

Guilt

There is a common moral compulsion to keep doing as much as you can to assuage an overwhelming sense of guilt. Guilt is a greedy emotion and is never satisfied. Guilt is usually misplaced – is it really your fault that you have a painful condition? Have you committed a moral crime by having a bit of downtime? Ironically, people who feel a lot of guilt shouldn't, and those who never feel it probably should.

Guilt is a sticky emotion that is hard to reason away. Sometimes we are brought up to feel guilty about everything, and certain religions are especially good at making people feel bad about themselves. As you are likely to feel guilty anyway, why not rebel a bit and just accept that you'll feel a bit of guilt, whatever you do. It's important to remember that it's just a feeling habit that usually doesn't belong.

Acceptance of pacing

Like 'pacing', 'acceptance' is a big bogey Marmite word. My suggestion is to deal with what is in front of you now, at this point, and leave the big questions to another day. I will come back to this later, but for now I want simply to say that pacing is not giving up or giving in.

I see pacing as making a positive step in adapting to change. If you have less pain as a result, it does not matter whether or not you accept things at this point. Just doing something about it is the most important thing – adapt first, then think about acceptance.

Fight or lose

The biggest myth is probably the idea that if you do not fight your condition, it will beat you. Trying hard is a good thing, but pushing so hard that it puts you in pain for several days metaphorically shoots you in the foot. The irony here is that the harder you fight, the worse pain gets. It is better to adopt the ancient Chinese idea that it is better to negotiate than to fight a losing battle.

I'll do less

Another myth is the idea that pacing means that you will do less, but the aim of pacing is actually to do more, not less. This is because you will prevent yourself having so many down days on which you do nothing. You will usually need to do less in the short term, but this will increase with time. Just like an injured athlete, it is important to work within limitations, not keep pushing through the limits and getting set back. The idea is to do less, but more often. In the end, you will do more, more often. I know this sounds boring and frustrating, but working within limits resets the pain circuits, which is really important.

Martyrdom

Putting everyone's needs before your own is a common reason for overdoing things. This is not to say that you should not help others, but doing everything for everyone will start to catch up with you. If you do not look after yourself, you risk not being able to help anyone.

Avoiding pain at all costs

There is also a myth that pacing means preventing pain at all costs. It doesn't. It is all about making choices, so you might sometimes choose to do something that causes more pain because doing it is more important than the pain. This is a very important idea to grasp. Managing pain is not really about pain – it is really about *managing life* so that you are in control, rather than the pain being in control. With limited resources, it is important to make better choices based on your values so that whatever you do is for the right reasons – for you. Think about a hangover: everyone knows that they 'chose' it, but no matter how bad the experience of the hangover, it is tempered by the happy memory of how you got it.

If I don't beat it, it'll beat me

This too is a common misconception. The trouble is that it is based on other situations where fighting leads to victory. I am not suggesting that you should not fight, but don't fight against yourself, which is what we are doing when we are so hard on ourselves.

What it means

I keep saying that pacing means this or that, but in fact it is not that sophisticated. It's just a few basic principles. Ultimately, the big idea is to improve choice. This is very important because many people are convinced that they do not have any.

The choice lies in *what* you choose to do and/or *how* you choose to do it. There are some simple techniques that you can apply to help with this, but ultimately pacing – or whatever you want to call it – is a mindset based on the question *What choice do I have?* It's not just about what you choose to do or how you choose to do it; it's also about how you choose to respond to those pesky 'yes, buts'.

There are two ideas that keep peeping their heads around the corner: the impact of stress on our ability to make decisions, and the need to be kind to ourselves. I will discuss these more later, but I just wanted to say hello to them here and make you aware that they are very important.

Summary

Pacing is simple. Dealing with the 'yes, buts' is the tricky bit. Ultimately, it is all about adapting to unwanted change by doing things differently, but we often don't want to admit that we need to.

5

Stress, the caveman's guide

Stress is caused by being here and wanting to be there.

Eckhart Tolle

In cowboy films, there is often someone flash in a top hat and waistcoat selling the elixir of life, the cure-all for everything from epilepsy to warts. Everyone knows that his product is a con, but he usually sells a few bottles to people drawn in by the patter. And who knows, the power of placebo can be astonishing – sometimes placebo wins over medicine when the two are tested against each other. I also heard of a man in Ireland who swore by the WD-40® household lubricant he put on his joints.

Obviously, we all want an easy answer, a magic cure for pain with no side effects that would also stave off other conditions. Sadly, there isn't one, but if you could distil it and bottle it, I am sure the real elixir of health would be one that cures stress.

Stress makes everything worse. It is a physical, physiological and psychological response to perceived threat. This simply means that if you feel threatened, you automatically become stressed. However, what counts as threat varies immensely, from life-threatening situations to the kitchen being untidy. Stress turns the turbo on, revs up the body systems and puts everything under a heavy load. It is a good thing in short bursts because it helps us to get out of trouble, meet deadlines and escape from marauding animals. This kind of stress is known as eustress. It is basically the caveman's healthy response to danger. I say 'caveman' because stress is an ancient response that we are hard-wired to produce when we feel threatened (Figure 5.1). Stress produces the fight or flight response, which basically means that when we are stressed, our inner caveman wants to hit someone or run away.

To fight or run away, our caveman needs to do a lot of things: there is a 100 per cent focus on the threat, his brain races to find a

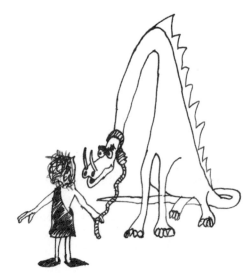

Figure 5.1 Our inner caveman, getting stressed trying to control something that has suddenly become a big threat. Threats come in all shapes and sizes – they don't have to look like a dinosaur. (Keen-minded readers and palaeontologists will rightly point out that *Homo sapiens* were not contemporaneous with dinosaurs.)

solution, his breathing quickens to get oxygen in, his heart races to get that oxygen via the blood to the muscles, stress hormones and adrenaline are released to steer energy to the muscles, the muscles tense, and emotions such as anger and fear rise quickly. This provides the ability to fight off the danger or run away. There is, however, a third option – to freeze – which tends to happen when the situation is overwhelming and he doesn't know what to do.

This is all great stuff and helps the caveman survive in his dangerous world full of life-threatening situations that often involve big pointy teeth or a genuine fear of starving to death. But the dangers we face in our modern world are usually very tame by comparison, yet we still have an ancient caveman, almost 'animal', nervous system that is trying to help us in a world it was not designed for. It is like having an overprotective friend who is with you all the time – he's short-tempered, is easily frightened, gets in fights, runs away a lot, wants to have sex with everyone and won't let you sleep if he thinks things aren't safe. Obviously, he needs managing.

The fight or flight stress response is a powerful primal response to danger that is sometimes useful, but is usually too powerful compared with the realities of modern life and out of proportion to reality. It's like having a Ferrari with the brakes and suspension of a mobility scooter. This can cause major issues with the kind of long-term stress that the caveman was not designed for, and this produces distress.

Distress

Distress occurs when the stress response stays switched on or all that stress energy has nowhere to go. Some people describe it as having a foot on the accelerator and the brake at the same time, revving hard but not going anywhere. And like a bridge, if you are under too much load for too long, something eventually gives. The bridge collapses at its weakest point, and so do people. Stress uses up vast quantities of energy, and if the stress continues people simply get worn out.

The effects of long-term stress add up: this is known as allostatic load. This can show as pain or fatigue, or the onset of a new condition. Allostatic load is simply the result of the stress-chemical-producing parts of the body (known as the hypothalamic–pituitary–adrenal axis) getting stuck on red alert. This can then go two ways: someone can be stressed all the time and get anxious seemingly over nothing, or they can become completely worn out and shut down, sometimes both.

One serious effect of high-level stress is known as post-traumatic stress disorder. This is where the system undergoes such a shock that it stays on red alert all the time. We are familiar with soldiers experiencing this, but childhood trauma affects untold thousands. In severe cases, you need to seek professional help through your doctor and access psychological and counselling services to help unpack the traumas safely.

Where is stress?

Ask someone where their stress is and they will usually point to their head. Contrary to popular belief, however, stress is located more in the body than the brain. It is the opposite of pain, which is more to do with the brain than the body. The clue lies in the way we talk about 'feeling stressed'. Stress is part mental – the brain fires the starting gun and decides whether you should be stressed – but the reality of stress is that it is mostly a physical experience.

Everyone experiences stress in different ways. It is important to know your own personal signs so that you can spot stress developing and do something about it. People are sometimes so used to being stressed that they do not realize they are – I call this 'stealth stress'. A good example is how lots of people have a condition called temporomandibular joint disorder, which causes pain in the jaw and face, and problems with chewing, but I would argue that in many cases this is a classic stress response rather than a condition in its own right.

It is also important to understand the difference between the difficulties caused by your condition and those caused by stress. Ultimately, as the person in the middle of all of this, you get both, but it helps to differentiate because we can also do something about stress separately from any condition we have. If you look at the effects of stress, you might just realize how big a deal this is as it can produce or contribute to, among other things, irritable bowel syndrome, lack of sleep, tense muscles, grinding teeth, reduced immune function and susceptibility to infections, anxiety, strong emotions, depression, headaches and inflammation. All these can make pain worse or complicate the picture, and although stress is not the only cause of these, it is certainly a major factor that tends to be ignored.

It is important to realize that it is not all about pain. This change in health status adds to the stress that has built up from daily life, the past and difficulties we have previously encountered. But stress tends not to get taken seriously. Personally, I think stress is a major health hazard, and that healthcare in the future needs to focus on it to a greater degree. Not as a sideline, but as a mainstream issue.

Stress and emotions

Emotions always accompany stress. Stress is produced as a simple response to threat, and then emotion colours it according to the situation. The bigger sister of emotions in the pain world seems to be fear, with its smaller siblings of anxiety, anger and frustration not far behind. Although anger and fear are the 'fight and flight' emotions, in my experience frustration is very often the first emotion people complain of, with anxiety a close runner-up. In reality, though, anxiety about what needs to be done may end up fuelling the frustration that drives people to keep on doing things despite the pain.

As emotions are part of the stress response, it is no surprise that they are also helpful if appropriate and short term, but unhelpful if they are inappropriate or disproportionate, or stay switched on for too long. The caveman is right to be frightened of the snake. In fact, his fear helps him avoid it, and he really does need to be afraid of poisonous snakes. But if he stays frightened of snakes when he knows there are none about, that will prevent him going out and will disturb his sleep. I hope you can see here parallels with anxiety over things that are unlikely to happen.

I like to invent new words. So, in the same way that we talk about 'eustress' and 'distress', maybe we could also have 'eumotions' and 'dismotions'. As with the stress picture, the 'eumotions' are useful to a point, but if they go on too long they start to trip us up and hold us back – that's the change from 'eu' to 'dis'.

Because stress acts as the foot pump for emotions, you will be more emotional when you are stressed. At this point, your emotions start to take over and distort your thinking. As we saw in the boom–bust cycle, we may become stressed that we will not finish a job, so then we become angry or frustrated or guilty, and this blinds us to common sense.

Common sense is a contentious issue. A wise man told me once that it was neither common nor sensible, and that has rattled around in my head ever since. The point with common sense is that it makes sense on your own terms. If you are desperate to do something, putting yourself in pain as a result seems fine, but it only seems sensible in the heat of the moment, within the time frame of doing the job. Look back in hindsight from the following day and you will realize that yesterday's logic does not make sense today. You perhaps got carried away with something that really was not so important.

There is a rule in therapy that we make the best choices we can at the time. Which is another way of saying that things make sense to us based on what we know and believe at the time. A change in what you know and believe will probably lead to different choices and a different kind of common sense. One major idea I want to introduce here is that we need to know more about ourselves. We need to be aware that stress and emotions distort our thinking and that it is good to know when to ignore ourselves.

Cumulative stress

Stress is not a one-off thing, but we often blame it on a single, trivial event like a ticking clock or someone who has said, 'You look well!' when we feel awful. Funnily enough, during group work over the years, I have had to disable quite a few clocks or put them outside because people cannot bear their 'deafening' sound; they say it winds them up. The point is that it is not the clock that is so stressful, but the build-up of everything else that is the real issue. Small events can be the 'straw that breaks the camel's back'.

Stress builds up. We all carry around a rucksack of our own challenges and stressors. Sometimes we call this our 'baggage'. Some people have more in their rucksack than others. Some rucksacks were filled up early in life and have been dragging their wearer down ever since. And some rucksacks have suddenly got heavier with the burden of chronic pain.

The point is that stress builds up, and it is the final small extra weight that shows how heavy the rucksack is. We cannot take everything out of our rucksack immediately, but we can usually make it a bit lighter. Even a small improvement helps because it is the excess baggage that is the issue. We need to reduce the weight in our rucksack a little or get better at carrying it.

In my teens I went through a phase of lugging rucksacks up hills for 'fun'. I suppose it was the only holiday available at the time, and my friends and I also hoped to meet unattached women who were heading the same way. Sadly, we didn't, but I do remember how miserable it was to lug that great weight around all day. I also remember the joy of taking the rucksack off at the end of our hikes and walking feeling almost weightless, like an astronaut. Just one less can of baked beans to carry seemed to be like losing a ton.

This links to one of my main themes: focus on the things you can change now rather than being overwhelmed by attempting to clear the whole rucksack. Even a small reduction in weight can make a disproportionately large difference. Maybe the relief comes from realizing that improvement is possible, that the load can be lessened, and that you are not so weak after all.

Stress and pain

Pain gets the blame for so much, but this is unfair and unhelpful because stress is often an invisible elephant in the room, standing beside the pain elephant. The stress elephant annoys the pain elephant but no one notices. Everyone tries to get rid of the pain elephant, but they won't succeed because the door is being blocked by the stress elephant, who is jammed in it.

Stress is everywhere in chronic pain. Anywhere you slice it, you find stress lurking. There is a strong stress response to pain, but it also relates to maintaining standards and worrying about what others think of you, about money, about the future, about relationships and about what the heck to do about your condition. If chronic pain were a stick of rock, it would have the word 'stress' running all the way through it. However, everyone understandably focuses on the pain and forgets that stress is at the centre of the pain experience. To go back to our pain knot analogy from Chapter 1, when you look closely at the knot, you will see that most of the strands have more to do with stress than pain. Some people say, 'If I didn't have the pain, I wouldn't have the stress', but as we can't immediately remove the pain, we need to reduce the stressors that are driving it.

From a caveman perspective, there is something very basic going on. The caveman needs to have all his faculties in top form so that he can compete in the 'survival of the fittest' competition that is pre-civilization life. No NHS or welfare state for him. So if he is under par for any reason, he is more vulnerable to attack and he needs stress to alert him to it. As there are more physical threats for our caveman, so stress kicks in more forcefully because life is more dangerous. These days, we are not at risk of dying by not being able to sprint away from a marauding sabre-toothed tiger, but we feel vulnerable just the same.

The pain–stress cycle

Pain is stressful, and stress winds up pain. Pain is accompanied by a stress response, but living with pain also creates lots of stress. This creates a catch-22 situation, a vicious cycle in which stress and pain feed off each other. And because, as I said above, we cannot instantly change the pain, we need to go round to the back door and deal with the stress instead, shrinking the stress elephant so that the door can be unblocked for the pain elephant.

Stress, together with all those bodily changes, heightened emotions and wonky thinking, is what happens when we think that something is a threat. So to reduce stress, we need to tackle the threat. We need to use practical means to reduce the threat itself wherever possible; see things positively or just more realistically; do things to calm down; and burn off the energy produced. I call this the '4 Ps' approach.

- Practical. Do what you can to reduce the cause in practical terms.
- Perception. See how you can think of the situation in a more realistic or more positive way, which also involves distracting your attention.
- Peace. Do things to feel calmer, such as using relaxation techniques.
- PE. Do something physical to burn off your excess energy.

Let me give you an example of where I didn't get this quite right but my wife showed me how it should have been done. One evening, we heard loud music coming from the nearby flats. I had a strong stress response; my wife stayed calm. Let's trace this through the 4 Ps.

Practical: I went round and banged on the door to tell them to turn it off. No one answered so I considered calling the police. I spoke to another neighbour who was as grumpy as me. My wife stayed calm and thought I was overreacting.

Perception: I was cross because I thought a bunch of louts had moved in, but my wife thought it was just a blip and they probably hadn't realized how loud they were being; she was sure it would finish soon. She accused me of being an old grump, which she thought was funny. I told her that I'd met the other neighbour, who was stressed too. This helped me to feel that I was being reasonable, but persuaded my wife that I really was an old grump. I tried to distract myself by disappearing into the study and writing something.

Peace: I should have played a relaxation CD. My wife meanwhile carried on watching something unchallenging on TV.

PE: I should have gone for a walk instead.

My wife's view was that the situation needed to be put in perspective. She thought, 'It's not late, so I'll give them an hour and then get stressed.' She also reminded me that I had banged on the wrong door and been shouted at by an even grumpier woman in curlers! This real-life example shows that not all options are appropriate and that it's good to run through your options first. It also shows how two people get stressed differently and choose to respond in different ways.

I am now going to pepper you with lots of suggestions that might help in such situations. On the basis of doing what you can rather than what you can't, see if any of these ideas appeal to you. This of course overlaps with other sections of the book, especially Chapters 6 and 11 on relaxation and coping.

- Do something, no matter how small, as this diverts the energy of stress into action and unloads the rucksack a little.
- Introduce an alternative perspective by identifying what you would say to a friend in the same situation.
- Do something immediately to slow your breathing down. As I say in Chapter 6 on relaxation, the brain thinks that slow breathing equals calm.
- Try to be realistic. For example, I find myself getting annoyed at busy airports, but that's what airports are supposed to be and I'm adding to it!
- Score your reaction out of ten compared with the reality of the situation. What could you do now to lower your reaction by one point or improve the reality by one point?
- Put things in context – what's the worst that could happen, what's the best, what's the most likely?

- What do others you know do in this situation? Do an Internet search for it.
- Distract yourself. Do something else that you can lose yourself in.
- Make practical plans. Focus on sorting what's bothering you rather than dwelling on your reaction to it.
- Have a positive piece of wisdom that you use as a motto – my dad's is 'worse things happen at sea'.
- Push the acupressure point for anxiety, which is in the dent on your wrist in line with your little finger.
- Focus beyond the situation you are facing. What will it be like when it's all over? Some people fill this out with: what will it look like, sound like, feel like and smell like? And while you are there, look back at how you will have overcome the situation.
- Talk to people. Everything is better if you share it, get others' input and talk through things. This ties in with my dad's other piece of advice: 'better out than in'!

Summary

Stress is a huge issue in chronic pain, but many people avoid looking at it because they think that it is a side issue. That if the pain went, so would stress. But this is unlikely because there is always stress in life.

There is also a perception that pain is pain, and that stress hints at something less physical. However, the reality is that pain is a complex experience which is certainly affected by issues such as stress. Ironically, though, stress is largely a physical experience. And if pain isn't changing right now, you need to make life better around it. Not only that, but if you reduce stress then, to throw all our metaphors in, generally the pain knot starts to unravel, the stress elephant shrinks out of the doorway, the camel's back gets better, the caveman relaxes and you might just find that your pain improves and you are not as stressed by what remains.

6

Relaxation

Tension is who you think you should be. Relaxation is who you are.

Chinese proverb

Relaxation is the fire extinguisher for stress. It slows things down, creates a gap between you and your fears, lowers blood pressure, provides respite, is something that you can do for yourself, creates the body's own painkillers (called endorphins), releases tension, reduces stress, breaks up pain, helps with sleep, is generally very nice, doesn't have side effects and is free. Over the years, many people have told me that learning to relax was the first big step that they made towards improving things. I'm a big fan; I hope you will be too.

For proper relaxation, three things need to come together: you need to feel safe, slow your breathing and have a focus. If you have not been able to relax in the past, it is probably because one element is missing. Often people take a few puffs of breath and say, 'See, it doesn't work!' So maybe we should add a fourth element: that you need to want to do it.

To cut to the chase, we should start with the simplest form of relaxation. All you need to do here is breathe more slowly than normal. Although this will work on its own, to do it properly you need to breathe in through your nose, let your tummy relax so you look fat and then breathe out through your mouth.

As you breathe out through your mouth, your tummy will naturally fall back. If you can't do the tummy thing straight away, just concentrate all your attention on your breathing in a relaxed, gentle way and eventually your tummy will join in. Some people find it hard to breathe in through the nose or out through the mouth, so should just use whatever route they can.

Sit in a chair and try this in whatever way works. The key thing here is to just focus on breathing, and to do it more slowly and more deliberately than usual. If you get anxious, try not to worry but just do what you can. You will find that this simple technique is helpful in many day-to-day situations when things are starting to get on top of you. It is also helpful when lying in bed trying to get to sleep – just rest your hands on your abdomen, focus on your breathing and close your eyes. Counting your breaths also helps with focusing.

Whenever you do a relaxation, it helps to go somewhere quiet where you will not be disturbed for a while – on its own this will be relaxing, but the relaxation practice will deepen this. In time you will find that you can practise relaxation, especially the simple breathing technique – to paraphrase an old advertising slogan for a certain brand of alcohol: you can learn to relax virtually anywhere at any time and in any place. But don't forget the obvious common-sense cautions. Don't practise relaxation when you are driving or operating heavy machinery, for example, and, after relaxation, make sure that you are awake enough to do these or similar tasks

The simple breathing technique is the cornerstone of all relaxation. It is also a good start for those who are anxious about switching off. If you feel worried about relaxing because it is a new idea or you do not want to let your guard drop, practise the breathing as though it is an exercise the physiotherapist has given you that you need to follow. With time, you will find that you feel more confident and that you start to let your eyes close.

Relaxation works because it is the opposite of stress. In stress, we focus on a threat, we feel unsafe and our breathing speeds up. During relaxation, we do the opposite, so the muscles relax and everything slows down. If you practise regularly, you will build a skill, or habit, called the relaxation response. This simply means that you will relax more quickly and easily over time. This is a great skill to have because many people say that they find it hard to relax when their pain is bad. The better you become at this technique, the easier it is to do even with bad pain. John in Hexham nods off the instant I say we are going to do a relaxation exercise – that's what I call a very well-developed relaxation response.

When we talk about relaxation, it is important to mention distraction. Here you turn your attention to other things such as hobbies and personal interests, and these will help you calm down and relax. Distractions are especially important if you are nervous about relaxation itself. It is really important to make sure that you spend time every day doing something that takes your mind off your worries.

People sometimes feel reluctant to practise relaxation because they feel too guilty to do it in case it looks like they are being lazy. I want to suggest, however, that relaxation is important therapy. It takes discipline to make sure you find time and do it, preferably at the same time every day. It takes effort and application to build a good relaxation response, but over time you will be pleased you have done it.

I cannot overstate the usefulness of relaxation. I have worked with a number of people who have reduced their medicine as they have become better at relaxation. Once you start to feel the benefits, you will probably wonder why you haven't been doing this for years.

And there are many sorts of relaxation and visualization to choose from – I have listed a few below, with a brief description of how to do them. You might also benefit from listening to pre-recorded relaxation from a CD or online source. Everyone is different, so you need to find one that suits you. The same applies to choosing the technique you respond best to – it's a personal thing.

Remember always to do relaxation in your own way. What you feel will vary from session to session, but the key is to keep at it. The more you do it, the more you will benefit. Make sure that you find a quiet place, turn off that pesky mobile and allow yourself to relax by recognizing that relaxation is a vital part of your pain management.

Relaxation techniques

Everyone is different and you need to find a relaxation technique that works for you. I would recommend that you do two ten-minute sessions every day. You may wish to do one session when you are in bed so that it helps you to fall asleep. You can, of course, do more if you wish, but here are some ideas for what to do.

Colour breathing

You can add to the simple breathing technique described above by adding colour. Think of a colour for calm and breathe it in. Then think of a colour for stress, breathe it out and see it float away from you like a vaping cloud. Do this for a while and then maybe breathe in a colour for comfort and visualize it going to a place where you feel pain. See it diluting the pain and then breathe out a colour you choose for pain.

This works very well if you like colour. Most people choose dark colours such as red and black for stress and pain, and lighter colours for the good things – calm and comfort. However, it doesn't matter which colours you use; they just need to work for you.

Fingers together

Just breathe slowly and put your fingers together. Focus on your fingertips one at a time and feel the pressure and warmth in detail. Then gently release the pressure between the touching fingertips, and maybe even separate them. Then slowly bring them back together, noticing everything in detail as you do it. This is an excellent, reassuring and practical way to calm down. It also involves a physical anchor, which many people find helpful.

Confusional technique

I mention this again in Chapter 7 on sleep. I call it my baked beans relaxation because I use the number 57. This technique helps to stop your mind racing. Breathe in and out as described above and settle in to a good slow rhythm. After a while, count up from 1 on the in-breath and down from 57 on the out-breath, so it will be 1-57, 2-56, 3-55 and so on.

Of course, if you are a maths genius, this will be too easy for you so you could use the alphabet instead: a-z, b-y, c-w . . . . Or you could count up from 26 and down from 34. Your numbers will then quickly cross over, which causes lots of 'fun'. Or you could count each way away from 27: 26-27-25-28-24-29. I think this is probably the hardest to do, even for mathematical types.

Favourite place

Slow your breathing and gradually relax. Think of a favourite place and describe it to yourself in terms of all the senses: what you can see, hear, feel, smell and taste. You can go wherever you want to, but just make sure that it is a place which is safe and has only positive memories for you.

The progressive autogenic technique

This sounds a bit of a mouthful, but 'autogenic' just refers to relaxation techniques that aim to control the body's underlying physiological processes; that is, its underlying functions. Ultimately, it's about harnessing the immense power of the mind to affect the body.

First, slow your breathing and focus on your head or legs. Then work up, or down, bit by bit – this is the 'progressive' bit. You need to say silently to yourself: 'My feet feel relaxed, my legs are getting heavy, my tummy feels warm, my arms feel heavy, my shoulders are relaxing, my jaw relaxes as I open my mouth.' Focus up and down your body several times as you breathe slowly. It helps to do things like unclench your hands and let your arms drop. Just keep going up and down in waves.

Mindfulness

Think of just sitting on a river bank watching the leaves and sticks flow past. The river is a metaphor for thinking and feeling – a stream of consciousness. In a mindfulness session you just observe what you notice happening, and step back from your normal ways of reacting and labelling things.

First settle down. Slow your breathing and notice everything in detail. Notice how you are breathing. Notice what is happening in your body when you breathe, and notice how long it takes to breathe in and out. Notice how you are sitting in your chair, and notice how you feel physically. Notice your feet on the floor; notice your hands and how they feel, how warm they are. Notice how you are thinking. Notice things as they occur. You could scan your body from head to toe, or toe to head, and notice what you notice, and then notice the next thing you notice. It's all about noticing.

Even if there seems to be nothing to notice, that is always still something. If you notice a sound, try to describe it to yourself without saying what it is. If you get annoyed, notice that you are annoyed, and notice the different components of being annoyed. Similarly, notice how you are feeling and describe everything to yourself as though you were telling someone else. Notice the details of things but try to put your judgement to one side. Carry on for as long as you want. If you find noticing yourself difficult, you can just visualize yourself watching a beautiful river and describe what you see.

Some people say that this sort of practice is like looking at the world through thick glass: you observe but don't get caught up in it. The idea is that it is important to be in the 'moment', experiencing things just as they actually *are* right now, rather than how you think they are or how you project them into the past and future. This is just like watching the river of life – things come and then they go.

Deeper relaxation with an 'anchor'

This is a counting-down relaxation with an 'anchor' when you are at your most relaxed. The anchor is simply putting your fingers together so that your body remembers what you are feeling. Once you have practised this repeatedly, you will have created a useful conditioned reflex of immediately feeling calm when you put your fingers together, which you can use when you need to feel calmer.

To do this exercise, simply breathe slowly again and let everything slow down. You can use different techniques here to settle down. One I like is to notice in detail everything about how you are sitting – how your hands are, how you are sitting in your chair, how your feet are resting on the ground.

Then count down slowly from whatever number you want – 10 is a good one. As you breathe in and breathe out, slowly count down. At each lower number, let yourself relax more deeply. In your head, say 'calmer' and 'calmer still' to yourself. You can also feel heavier or warmer, or feel a wave of ease moving up and down your body. Let all your muscles relax, feel like you are made of lead and see your worries going over the horizon. Keep counting down, and at zero create a picture of whatever you want – maybe a favourite scene, maybe just a colour, maybe just feeling calmer and calmer, heavier and heavier, more and more switched off. At some point when you are feeling at your best, put your thumb and forefinger together, just for 30 seconds to a minute, and then release them.

When you are ready start to count yourself back up to 10, feeling more and more awake as you count up.

Detailed memories

Again, settle in to your breathing. Let everything slow down and relax. Once you are relaxed, you can start to answer some questions that you may wish to set yourself. For example, can you name all of your cousins? What was the first record that you bought? Who were your friends at primary school and what were their nicknames? What was the first address you lived at? What was the colour of the front door? What was each room like? What was the garden like? If you were going to a certain place, how many left turns would there be and what landmarks would you go past? If a tourist was visiting the area, where would you tell them to go? When were you last there? What did you have for tea two evenings ago? When did you last see some blue sky? Or notice a strange cloud? A classic that many people use is to take themselves through everything that happened on a good holiday in minute detail – who was in front of you in the queue for check-in? What was your seat number? . . .

Summary

The techniques listed here are just tasters to use to see how self-directed relaxation works for you. I can nearly always knock myself out with my baked beans technique, but if I need a bit more I play about with the others. They are all safe because you are in charge and can stop any time you want. And remember to enjoy your relaxation.

Learning to relax is the Swiss army knife for life with pain – it has something to help in every situation.

7

Sleep

Sleep is the golden chain that ties health and our bodies together.

Thomas Dekker, *The Gull's Hornbook*, 1609

When I ask about sleep, most people with chronic pain look at me quizzically and say, 'What's that?' In fact, it's amazing how many people with chronic pain also have poor-quality sleep. Sleep is a major contributor to health issues. Like stress, it is often considered to be a secondary issue in relation to pain, but it is a core component that can explain much of a person's situation.

I am not saying that poor sleep is the only factor, but if the fittest people in the world slept badly, it would soon begin to take a toll on their health and quality of life. At the very least, they would be tired and sensitive, but they would probably soon develop other conditions. I mentioned this earlier, but it's worth repeating: a doctor friend told me that when she was training in the 1980s, when junior doctors had exceptionally long shifts, some started to develop fatigue and strange aches and pains that could not be explained – a bit like some chronic conditions.

Poor sleep is probably the third elephant that enters the room after pain and stress. In a way, these are all related. Life with pain is stressful, stress winds up pain, and stress makes sleep harder. Improving sleep is obviously vital in helping to unravel the knot.

Improving sleep is easier said than done, but for fun I wanted to share a quip from comedian W. C. Fields, who said that the best way to deal with poor sleep is to get lots of it. I couldn't agree more, because this would break the cycle of knowing that you won't sleep. Quite how you do this is the tricky bit that he missed out. But when you understand what is happening with sleep, there are a few surprisingly simple things that can make a big difference.

Two basic approaches can improve sleep. The first is a bit bossy; this is called sleep hygiene, and it consists of a set of 'rules' that make sleep more likely. The second strategy involves slowing a racing mind that is often spinning like a twin-tub washing machine at two in the morning.

But first a few sleep facts. Sleep comes in cycles that last approximately 90 minutes. In theory, we go through a number of stages:

- light sleep (when you are easily woken by the cat);
- non-rapid eye movement (non-REM) sleep (deepening to deepest sleep when bombing by the cat wouldn't wake you);
- REM sleep (coming back up, which is when you dream);
- light sleep (when you might wake briefly and go to the loo or push the cat off your head).

Contrary to popular belief, it is normal to wake a few times in the night. The trouble is that some people then find they stay awake, and this is when the mind starts to race like a hamster on a wheel.

The amount of sleep needed varies from person to person. Some need ten hours while others get away with much less. The key to understanding your need is whether you feel tired in the day. If you do and it is not just boredom, you are not, generally speaking, getting enough sleep.

The nature of sleep means that we do not really know how well we have slept. I recently woke and then woke again, apparently the next minute. I thought I was having a terrible night, but when I looked at the clock it was actually two hours later.

Some people find it useful to use sleep apps so that they can measure how they do actually sleep. This is especially important to deal with some of the myths people build around sleep. Margaret in Hexham said: 'With my condition, you don't get deep sleep.' But when she tried a sleep app, she discovered that she did actually go into deep sleep. I hoped that this shattered her view of her situation – in a good way. This is of relevance because some studies show that how people think they have slept has a direct effect on how tired they feel the next day.

The idea that we should sleep in a block is not set in stone either. In medieval times, when everyone slept in the same room, the night was often a game of two halves with people sleeping, then socializing, then sleeping again. Finally, it is useful to distinguish between a sleep and a nap, and, for that matter, a power nap. The key idea is that a sleep is a cycle involving all the stages. If you sleep for only a bit of the cycle and then wake, you will often feel really groggy. A power nap can help, but remember that sleeping in the day can eat into sleeping at night.

Sleep hygiene

Sleep hygiene is not about having a wash before you go to bed; it's more to do with the rules that make it most likely you will sleep well. There is nothing remarkably new about this because it is all rooted in what we all did when we were little.

The key idea is to treat yourself like a small child. Children need to learn how to sleep, or rather they need repeats of the same elements so that they learn the habit of sleep. The key ideas are a bedtime routine, a set bedtime and getting-up time, a story and a warm, safe place with low lighting. Basically, that is what we also need to do as adults if we have got out of the habit of good sleep.

The (bossy) rules are as follows.

- Have a set bedtime and a getting-up time.
- Don't have a TV or mobile phone in the bedroom – a radio is fine, though.
- Don't eat too near to bedtime.
- Reduce your caffeine intake, especially after midday, and certainly don't drink any caffeine drinks in the middle of the night.
- Have a bedtime routine: maybe have a warm bath and turn the lights off one at a time.
- Use the bedroom only for sleep – no work or checking your mobile.
- Get outside during the day. Daylight reinforces the body clock because, like flowers, we follow the light.
- Don't sleep during the day, especially if you are unable to sleep at night.
- Go to bed before midnight.

In ancient times, many sleep-promoting features were inherent in life. There was no television, no artificial light, no smartphones or Facebook to get caught up in, a dearth of coffee shops, in fact no coffee at all. In a way, sleep hygiene takes us back to the basics that make sleep more likely.

I know it all sounds a bit bossy, but it's bossy in a good way. If you follow these rules, sleep is more likely. And that's half the battle. The rest of the battle is dealing with waking in the middle of the night, or not getting to sleep in the first place.

Taming the hamsters

When we are up and about during the day, our attention is split between many and various things, but at night anything that pops up can be focused on by 100 per cent of our attention. Not only that, but at night we are obviously tired, and in caveman terms sleep is also when you feel vulnerable. That is why you need to feel safe so that you can switch off and let your guard drop. Sleep is the opposite of stress, so if you are stressed sleep will be hard.

If you are lying awake in the middle of the night, it's easy for the mind to lock on to anything that crops up, and then it starts to race like a hamster on a wheel. Throw a problem onto a hamster wheel and it soon grows into a big worry. To mix in another metaphor, we make mountains out of molehills when we pay them too much attention.

There are three main concerns that leap onto the hamster wheel that keep people awake at night. First, when we cannot sleep we start to think about this and become desperate to go to sleep. But the more desperate we get, the more stressed we get, and so we stay awake.

Second, when an issue drops in to the mind, it quickly gets revved up, but trying to solve something with too much attention rarely works. We often get caught up in 'what if' and tend to find more questions than solutions. So again we get stressed and stay awake.

Finally, pain is often awful in the middle of the night because we have too much attention available with which to notice it. All that attention also goes into thinking about the pain (remember primary and secondary suffering in Chapter 2). Feeling more pain combined with all the worries about it creates heaps of stress that, you've guessed it, keeps you awake. So when you are feeling like this, it is usually impossible to get comfortable and drift off.

Slowing the racing mind

The fuel for all of these night-time difficulties is attention. It is a particular kind of attention in which we are tired and vulnerable so we focus too much, zoom in on the negative and are generally not able to put things in context or think in a straight line.

The way to improve things is to reduce attention, refocus the mind and thereby calm down and go to sleep. It is a good idea to develop a plan for doing this. Having a plan means that you do not have to reinvent the wheel every night. If it works, it also becomes the kind of familiar reassuring pattern that promotes sleep.

Here's one suggestion for your plan: do three things – get up, calm down, and go back to bed and relax. Getting up acts like pressing a reset button. However, it is important not wake up too much. One lady I worked with used to get up and do the housework. Not surprisingly, she wasn't able to get back to sleep. The idea is to get up and be a low-light zombie for a while. Maybe read a little – but not a page-turner or a horror story – maybe do a few stretches, a puzzle or whatever it takes to divert enough attention so your mind can start to calm down. The low light is important because bright light will wake you.

Once you have settled, you can move back to bed and try a few closed eye relaxations. The key for any night-time relaxation is to do something that occupies the ground between being interesting enough to take your attention, but not important enough to make you stay frantically awake to get it right. Here are a few suggestions.

- Count up from 1 and down from 57, alternating with each breath. This is an excellent way to get the mind busy doing something unimportant.
- Think of a holiday and remember its boring details: where you parked, where you sat on the plane and so on.
- Plan in detail how you would completely redecorate your house.

A clever member of one of my recent groups thought that his get-to-sleep challenge would be to remember all the moons in the solar system – apparently there are more than 50. Maybe he was just showing off, but if it gets him to sleep I really don't mind.

Relaxations (see also Chapter 6) can involve a favourite place or a pleasant focus on exactly what is happening with all your body parts: my right hand is sinking into the duvet, my legs are relaxing, my breathing is slowing, I can hear the cat purring, and so on.

Another classic strategy that ties in with the world of being positive is to review your day and think of ten good things about it. Then remember each one in detail in terms of what it looked like, felt like, smelt like and sounded like. It is unlikely you will get to ten because you will probably fall asleep trying.

Sleep often occurs when we stop trying too hard. Nigel told me that he tossed and turned until 5.30 in the morning. At this point he thought, 'I give up' and promptly fell asleep. The moral: give up trying too hard to sleep.

Summary

The sleep hygiene items are important because they retrain us in the same way we were trained as little children. Sleep is the opposite of stress, so anything we can do to reduce the stress surrounding sleep helps immensely. If you give up trying so hard, you will fall asleep. Funnily enough, if you try to stay awake, you will probably do the opposite!

8

Flare-ups

This too will pass.

Medieval Persian proverb

For most people, chronic pain is a roller coaster of ever-present pain with good days, bad days and flare-ups. All these affect us, but flare-ups cause the most upset.

Flare-ups are periods when pain is at its worst. They can last anything from days to weeks or even months. A 'flare-up' is something that lasts for a while and then settles; it does not mean pain that is 'always in flare-up' or something that strikes every few hours. Everyone is different and will have a unique experience of a flare-up.

I think of a flare-up as being akin to what happens at an oil refinery. When I see a glow in the sky over the refinery near my home, I know that they have too much gas in the system and need to burn it off. During this period, they will need to operate the refinery differently until the excess gas has been removed. It is the same with pain. The flare-up is a temporary period in which we need to reduce the load on the system by doing things differently. If we do not do this, the flare-up might last longer than it should. Imagine what would happen at the oil refinery if they did not bother to respond to the roaring 30-metre flame coming out of the chimney.

Setbacks

While we are talking about flare-ups, it's helpful to consider their cousin – the setback. A setback occurs when everything you are facing in life uses up all your coping capacity. It happens when you have been under a huge amount stress, when you've 'had it up to here' and there is not much left to cope with anything else. This is important because how well you cope is ultimately more important than the pain 'itself'.

If you are busy coping with everything else, you might not have the time or inclination to follow a pain management routine. This could be one reason for all the 'yes, buts' we talked about in Chapter 4. So you can see how a setback could easily lead to a flare-up. You can also see that if you are regularly 'up to here', flare-ups will happen more easily. And with chronic pain, there are many people who are 'up to here' most of the time. That's why stress and coping are so important.

PANTS

Going back to flare-ups, I see them as a compressed and magnified version of day-to-day life with chronic pain in which symptoms, worries, unhelpful thinking and stress chase each other around in an exhausting cycle. I like to describe this as the PANTS cycle (Figure 8.1).

The cycle can start at any point. More pain (P), for example, leads us to ask (A) a series of difficult questions, such as, 'How long will it last?' We then begin to think negatively (NT) about this – that it might never go away, for example. This in turn leads to stress (S), which winds pain up. In the middle of this sit our emotions, which become more negatively affected the more we go round the cycle.

One of the classic emotions traced out in the PANTS cycle is the simple wish for the pain to go away, quickly. This is only natural,

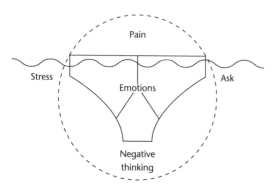

Figure 8.1 The PANTS cycle

but if we are desperate for the pain to go, we will become disappointed if it doesn't go immediately, and anxious about how long it will take. This stirs up stress, which revs up the whole cycle. This is a bit like the situation for sleep that I described in Chapter 7: the harder we try, the more desperate we get, the harder pain is to cope with and the longer it hangs around for.

An iceberg of pain

The PANTS cycle can also be drawn as an iceberg to describe life with pain. Even when pain is at manageable levels, there can be anxiety, negative thinking and stress whirring away out of sight beneath the surface of the water. A flare-up can occur when all the other issues surface. The pain at the tip of the iceberg is the bit that people can see and monitor, but most of what is going on usually lies under the surface.

Managing flare-ups

The best way to manage a flare-up is to prevent it in the first place by following the suggestions outlined in this book, but even if you are a black belt ninja in pain management, flare-ups are an inevitable part of life with a chronic condition. The good news is that we can take action to make flare-ups less likely and to reduce their effect when they do strike.

At its simplest, a flare-up occurs when we are overloaded, so the best response to a flare-up is to reduce the load for a while so we can return to our baseline as soon as possible. Reducing load means resting more, reducing stress and cutting down on commitments. Another way of seeing this is in terms of a fuel tank: a flare-up occurs when we are running on empty, so we need to freewheel a bit and refuel.

A natural response to flare-up is an urgent need to get rid of pain, but when pain does not go when we hope it will, desperation sets in. This creates stress that winds up the whole situation you are trying to damp down. The best response is to try to accept the situation, stay calm and know that things will improve in the usual time. I know this is hard, but it is important to try.

Shrinking your PANTS

A good structure for improving a flare-up, and for that matter life with pain in general, is to pick apart the PANTS cycle, shrink it and put the brakes on. Revisiting the cycle, let's look at improving each aspect.

Pain

During a flare-up, pain is often slow to respond to our attempts to get rid of it. It will settle, but it is hard to be convinced that it will. It is still important to do whatever you can to reduce pain for two reasons. First, physically, you can gain some relief, and the sooner you start a pain-relieving strategy, the better, even if your tactics are not having immediate effects. Second, psychologically, having something to do reduces the feeling of being a helpless bystander.

In a flare-up, it is time to get out whatever helps, even if only in small amounts. There is unfortunately no magic wonder gadget that we can use. Some people find TENS machines useful, many find heat or cold helpful, most people like warm baths, and everyone benefits from the right sort of chair. From experience, one of the best 'gadgets' is any portable device that will play music to help change a person's mood quickly. Music can be really helpful to motivate and soothe. Interestingly, the only bit of 'homework' that I can ever get people to do is to choose their *Desert Island Discs* to help their pain.

Ask

We can respond to the anxious questions in our heads – What caused this? How long will this last? What can I do? – in a more positive and realistic way. The experience of flare-ups in the past will have provided a good deal of knowledge, but that can be easily forgotten. This is why it is important to pay attention and even write things down so that a flare-up is not a surprising new experience every time.

A helpful response might be: 'There will be a reason for this flare-up, but I shouldn't beat myself up if I can't work it out now.' 'It will probably last as long as it did last time.' 'If it feels the same as before, then it will settle like it did before, and I'm unlikely to get stuck like this. But I know it's easy to think that, so I'll need to make practical changes for now to reduce stress. And if I'm not better in the usual time, I'll see the doctor.'

Negative thinking

When we feel brought down with pain or fatigue, it is natural to flip into negative thinking. Put simply, this is thinking that does not help because it is pessimistic and unrealistic. This means that it is easy to think pain will go on forever, that nothing will help and that you are a bad person for having it.

It is good to know your thinking habits so that you can catch yourself out and realize that thinking in a flare-up distorts reality and gives a false impression of what is really going on. One of the best ways of arguing with yourself is the reality test where you compare reaction with reality – this is described in Chapter 5. In this way, you can spot yourself being negative and then try to ignore yourself.

Some people emphasize that we need to be positive, but I would like to encourage realism. This is because being positive and thinking that pain will improve more quickly than it can inevitably leads to disappointment. Maybe the best combination is to be realistic with a hint of optimism.

Stress

Stress runs through this book like the writing inside a stick of rock. It is the reaction we have when we sense threat, and this piles high in a flare-up. Here stress is at the epicentre because it acts as the foot pump for emotions, wonky thinking and more pain. To add to the situation, many people feel depressed, anxious, frustrated, angry and guilty. These feelings pass in time, but when you are in the grip of them, it is hard even to imagine that things will improve. But happily they do.

In a flare-up, it is important to remove as many pressures as possible. That might mean cancelling a few commitments – tricky, but sometimes managing your flare-up is more important than making other people happy. Practise relaxation like it is going out of fashion. Do it a lot. It is hard work, but the effort you put in may help to take away the guilt that you are relaxing. Relaxation done properly is not swanning about or being lazy; it takes effort and discipline.

Emotions

It is hard and unhelpful to switch off all your emotions. You still need to have them and be allowed to have them. But if you experience difficult emotions, it is invariably better if you talk about how you feel.

Isolation is a big issue with a flare-up, so it is important to tell people how you are feeling. A person in pain often looks like a person who is cross with you, so it is helpful to be able to tell those you know and love that it is the pain that's making you grumpy, not them.

Know what your pain means

The standard reaction to pain is fear. This, of course, makes sense in acute pain, but in chronic pain we have to step back and realize the status of the pain we feel. If your pain is not related to new damage, it is time to rethink what it means. For example, many people's pain increases when the weather changes – so in a way it is just a signal that the weather has changed, and realizing this will help them react to it differently. As described in Chapter 2, it is worth considering (and checking with your clinicians) what your pain actually means, as well as the idea that hurt does not always equal harm. Sometimes pain is simply a sign of overload.

Planning

During a flare-up, when emotions are stronger than normal, it is hard to remember, concentrate or sometimes even think in a straight line. Even though you've been there and got the T-shirt a hundred times, it often feels like a new experience and that you need to find out what helps, and reinvent the wheel, every time. This is why it is important to make a note of what happens when you have a flare-up and build a plan so that you are prepared. Knowing what you are dealing with, and knowing what to do, reduces mystery, fear and stress – essential in dealing with pain.

The key to flare-up plans is not to focus too closely on the pain. You will know by now that focusing on pain makes it worse, so instead the emphasis should be on all the surrounding factors that make pain worse or harder to cope with. For some, creating a flare-up plan is about creating a plan or tick list to follow faithfully, whereas others just benefit from kicking ideas about and working out from that what they need.

A mnemonic can help us remember a good approach and also provides a bit of fun. Many of us already know the classic mnemonic RICE – rest, ice, compression, elevation – that reminds us what to do for inflammation after injury. That is a physical situation, but anything for chronic pain needs to mix physical, emotional and social factors. The key is to reduce the load for the short term to help us feel better and ensure that the flare-up passes as quickly as possible.

I've written a list (below) of the wide-ranging elements that can make up a plan. There are too many to make up a nifty mnemonic, although you could try.

- Tell someone. This is a surprising entry but it is what most people admit they never do.
- Ask for help. Counterintuitively, this can increase independence, not limit it.
- Stop saying 'Sorry'.
- Attitude. A realistic calm attitude helps, maybe remembering 'this too will pass'.
- Rest more than usual. A flare-up is your body shouting for a rest.
- Relax. Practise relaxation like it's going out of fashion!
- Distract yourself. Lose yourself in engrossing hobbies or interests.
- Gadgets. Use anything (safe and legal) that provides comfort and relief.
- Prioritize. Focus on what is most important while you have limited energy.
- Structure. A plan for the day will help to ensure that you get the right balance between work, rest and play.
- Therapy. Enlist some outside help – acupuncture, osteopathy, massage, or whatever attracts you.
- Endorphins. These are the body's home-made, self-regulating

opiates (painkillers) and are produced when we are enjoying ourselves. So don't forget to let yourself enjoy things and laugh.

- Awareness. Be aware that how you see the world will be distorted and negative during flare-ups.
- Knowledge. Know what normally happens in a flare-up, what helps, what doesn't, how long it normally lasts and how you think.
- Medical help. If the pain is different from normal or lasts longer, or if you have questions about your medicines, arrange to see your doctor.

I suggest that you pick out three or four essential items and make a word if you can. TARPs works well, which stands for: Tell, Ask, Relax, Prioritize, Structure. But obviously you don't need to make a word, just pick out what appeals to you. Or you could focus on aspects of the PANTS cycle. The main thing is to do something positive in response to flare-ups.

Summary

Flare-ups are short, compressed and very unpleasant versions of the daily experience of chronic pain. The usual cycle of stress and pain (PANTS) spins faster than normal and can drag us down in to a nasty mix of thoughts, feelings and experiences. The key to managing a flare-up is to radically reduce load in the short term.

The cause of flare-ups can be a mystery, but whatever causes them, they happen when we are overloaded in one way or another. The best way to manage a flare-up is to prevent it in the first place, but this is not always possible. Therefore we need to reduce the likelihood and duration of flare-ups by reducing load in all aspects of our lives. This means not living at 100 per cent of capacity, and assessing the balance between the 'fillers' and 'drainers' (for more on these, see Chapter 10).

The most important thing to do during a flare-up is to reduce your load so that you can recover as quickly as possible. In fact, reducing load is one of the main themes of pain management.

9

Food

Let food be your medicine and medicine be your food.

Hippocrates

Coal, wood, peat and small twigs are all fuel of a kind, but you would not put them in your car. If you tried it, you would get very strange looks at the petrol station and the car would conk out immediately.

It seems that we are good at putting the right fuel in our cars, but not so good at putting the right fuel in our stomachs. Part of what we need to remember is that the stomach is a very old bit of kit that struggles to deal with the onslaught that a modern diet throws at it. Finding the right diet to help with pain is like trying to nail a jelly to the wall – it's tricky. According to reports of 'studies', what kills you one week might save you the next, so it is hard to work out what to do. Regardless of the latest new superfood fad, what is certain is that what you eat and drink makes a big difference to your health.

One of the recurring themes in chronic pain is that everyone is different. This explains why it is hard to have detailed rules that apply to everyone. We have different food cultures and different genes, and most importantly our guts have different histories. A food that one person enjoys might not be tolerated by another. This all points to the fact that we first need general guidelines and then need to find our own unique approach.

The first and simplest reason that healthy eating is vital for living with pain is that it improves general health. Weight is an obvious factor because weighing more puts extra load on the joints that can make pain worse and make everything harder to do. Not surprisingly, losing weight often improves pain. The weight/fitness issue can be tricky, especially when a medicine has the adverse effect of adding weight and pain makes it hard to be active – hence it is very important to look at diet.

Many people turn to comfort eating. We naturally seek comfort when there is an upset in life, and if this does not come from other people in the amount we need, we may end up seeking comfort in fatty or sugary foods that pile on the pounds. Food is ultimately an emotional issue. Losing weight just by changing one's diet is only half the battle; the really important bit is to address the underlying emotional issues. Self-image is important here because many people have low self-esteem and losing weight could boost their confidence; however, the low mood resulting from low self-esteem and pain might prevent them believing that positive change is possible. If you have a very difficult relationship with food, it is important to seek professional help.

Another thorny issue relating to food that tends to produce a mixed reception, being derided by some, is the idea that some foods 'disagree' with us. That's a simple way of saying that there are foods that we are intolerant of. Intolerance is different from allergy, in which the reaction is quick, more severe, more noticeable and results from a particular pathway of reactions in the body. With intolerance, symptoms can rumble away in the background and not be at all obvious. An intolerance can, however, activate an inflammatory response and increase pain, even if it is not obvious what the root cause is. Some people dismiss this idea, but the message here is probably that if you find your pain worsens with a particular food and you benefit from cutting it out, that's all the evidence you need.

The major food groups relating to intolerance are wheat and dairy products, and more 'modern' foods that seem to affect many people. Mass-produced bread is often made from finely ground flour that our gut finds hard to deal with, and many people lack the enzyme that digests the milk sugar lactose, so tend to be lactose intolerant. If you feel one of these foods is affecting you, try cutting it out for a while and see whether you feel better. Then reintroduce it and see if you feel worse again; this can help identify trouble-makers. Anything can potentially be a problem. Some individuals find citrus foods make their arthritis worse, and others cut out the 'deadly nightshade' family of vegetables that includes tomatoes, peppers and onions.

Baddies

Some foods and drinks are just plain bad for us. We all know that we should not eat too much fat or sugar, but a little bit of what you fancy is often considered to be good for you. I believe, however, that some foodstuffs should be entirely avoided. These include highly processed convenience foods that are often packed full of preservatives and 'E numbers'. It is difficult to identify which of these are harmless and which, such as artificial sweeteners and colourings, could potentially affect health. But it is better to avoid or reduce these in favour of more natural products cooked from fresh; that way you know what is in what you are eating. Generally speaking, the further away something is from its original form or appearance, the more it has been processed.

Our guts evolved at a time when we were free-roaming and eating anything that came our way. At that point, everything was obviously organic and nothing was made in a factory. So, from a common-sense point of view, we can appreciate that our stomach is not designed to deal with foodstuffs and additives that have only existed for the last few decades. If our caveman was at the super-market, he would definitely be in the organic section.

Caffeine bingo

Caffeine is a chemical that is found in coffee, tea, chocolate and many fizzy drinks. It is also used in some medicines. It stimulates the nervous system, revs everything up and keeps us awake – which is why we like it. It is generally considered safe but, like everything, moderation is the name of the game.

It is funny how coffee in particular has become trendy, with people carrying small buckets of the stuff around town almost as fashion accessories – possibly as part of the 'must be busy' mindset. But there are also certain brands of fizzy, caffeine-filled, sugar-saturated drinks that many take everywhere. My group sessions are often accompanied by a grand display of such items. One of my simple goals in a course is to turn all the orange-, black- and blue-coloured liquids into water – almost the opposite of the Biblical water-into-wine miracle.

The trouble with caffeine is that if you have too much, you will be overstimulated. It can put you on a kind of wide-eyed red alert that you might just come to accept is normal. Not surprisingly, this can produce greater anxiety and worsen sleep. Many of us seem to use coffee as a strange mix of stimulating comfort, but drinking a lot can create a kind of empty energy and make you feel anxious – completely the opposite of comforting. It is good to be awake, but not too awake. Lots of people need a kick-start in the morning, but if you keep being kick-started all day, this will start to backfire.

Asking people about their caffeine intake is really effective because it identifies a quick and really beneficial lifestyle change that can be made. I call this caffeine bingo because it is simple and straightforward to do and often an easy win. Much of pain management can seem a bit subtle, but the need to drink less coffee is easy to grasp. In a previous chapter, I mentioned a grumpy lady with a 25-a-day coffee habit that she decided to change. Replacing the coffee with hot water and herbal tea meant that she slept better and her pain improved. Reducing caffeine is not rocket science, but it will make you feel that you are no longer sitting on one (Figure 9.1).

Steve, who lived in the Scottish Borders, was having a terrible time with stress and pain. He had begged for more pain medicine

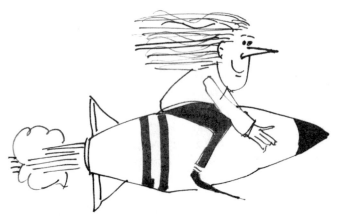

Figure 9.1 The caffeine rocket

so that he could sleep but he was on the maximum doses of every-thing. He was desperate for something he could do. When we talked, he admitted that he drank a lot of coffee, in his words 'just to keep going', so we looked at ways of reducing this. After a month, Steve said he was not noticing any difference, but I encouraged him to persevere. After two months of drinking less coffee, he came in grinning and saying 'You were right'. It didn't solve everything, but it reduced the hyperalert stressed feeling, and also gave him hope that things could improve, which is always very important.

It is not only the coffee, but also what you put into it that is important. One lady told me she had 30 cups a day, each with milk and three sugars. That's 30 teaspoons of sugar a day – a small mountain that is around three to five times the recommended daily intake of sugar from all the food we eat.

Goodies

Since everyone is different, it is hard to say exactly what we should have more of. Two simple ideas are to drink more water and eat more slowly so that you enjoy your food. This also helps the stomach, which works best when it is relaxed.

Eating more 'greens' seems to be important too, and washing fruit and vegetables removes potentially harmful chemicals.

Low glycaemic index (GI) foods such as porridge release energy gradually over a while rather than producing the sugar rush of high-GI foods, such as sugary breakfast cereals, chocolate and white bread. A simple change is to have brown rice instead of white.

The diet of choice seems to be the Mediterranean diet, which contains high quantities of olive oil, fruit, vegetables, oily fish, and so on. All the dietary advice I have looked at seems to have a similar message: more fruit and veg, more omega 3 oils (oily fish) and lean protein, and fewer heavy, fatty foods such as red meat and fried foods. Some sources say to cut out 'beige food', which is a nice way of saying that too many chips, biscuits and bread are not so good for us.

Some spices are said to help with inflammation, the favourites being ginger and turmeric. These can be added to cooking and even made into tea.

Our gut sometimes needs a bit of help to restore the balance of the bacteria that help to digest food and influence our immune systems. Some individuals take probiotics or traditional, naturally fermented foods such as kefir, kombucha, sauerkraut and live yoghurt.

Taking supplements is an area that is widely debated. In theory, we should get all our nutrition from our food, but modern diets and guts that do not work perfectly means that we sometimes lack some nutrients. The general thinking is that supplements should not replace natural food, but sometimes we need a little bit of help.

A big debate rages about organic food. Obviously, you need to make your own mind up, but think about where our caveman might shop . . .

Practical advice

Many people with chronic pain complain that cooking takes too much effort. The best practical advice I have come across is to batch-cook soups and stews that can be frozen so there is always a good healthy meal available. This also means that you achieve more with less, which is always good in pain management.

First and foremost, if you have been told to follow a special diet for medical reasons, don't change it. And in the same way that I keep suggesting that you should check medical issues with a clinician, you may need to check special dietary issues with, for example, a dietitian or a nutritionist. An extra bit of specialist nutritional help could be very useful.

It is crucial to make sure that you have the right nutrition to function properly. Make sure that you eat enough, and be aware of the effects of unhealthy foodstuffs.

Summary

I am not a dietitian or a nutritionist, and I suspect that you aren't either, but we all make decisions about our diet. Therefore it makes sense to look at some of the important ideas and identify simple ways in which to steer the diet ship better and make healthier choices.

It is hard to recommend one way of doing this because everyone is different. However, there are some important things that we can do to make a difference. One simple message is to eat less rubbish – you wouldn't put low-grade fuel in your car, so why put it in your body?

Eating better is far more important than many people think.

10

Life balance

All work and no play makes Jack a dull boy.

Old European proverb

Some ideas are much older than you might think. As far back as the seventeenth century, and probably earlier, when most of the population worked in the fields, they were talking about the balance between work and life. Someone somewhere came up with a fantastic bit of wisdom: all work and no play makes Jack a dull boy. For our times, this could be reworked as: all work and no play makes Jack an ill boy.

It can go the other way too. If Jack is forced out of work, then all play and no work will also upset Jack. More time on Jack's hands may mean that he becomes anxious, bored and embarrassed about justifying his existence; so he then fills his time up with 'jobs', so much so that he reverts to all work and no play. Either way, poor Jack is in trouble!

Finding the right balance in life is important for everyone, but, sadly, most of us get it wrong. It is absolutely fine and quite normal to be out of balance if it shows as only a little stress, but in the long term the stakes can be high. In Japan, they have a chilling concept – *karoshi* – which means death from overwork. I'm not suggesting this will happen to anyone, but it highlights the fact that long-term imbalance is a concern. If you are living with a chronic condition, the imbalance will show as an increased number of symptoms.

It is useful to clarify here that when I use the word 'work', I mean jobs and tasks, either paid or unpaid. We talk of 'going to work', but work is work regardless of the location. The advantage of paid work is that there is usually a clear structure and differentiation between being at work and then finishing. Unfortunately, modern technology means that work often follows people home. Phones that are still pinging at 10 p.m. means that many people are at work all day. This blurs the line between work and home, which is bound to create an unhealthy balance.

Unless you love doing it, 'work' is anything you have to do. It includes housework (the clue is in the word), DIY and other duties. Work also involves worrying about work. I'm writing this after a run to the recycling centre and some household chores, which to me are just as 'worky' as going to work on a Monday morning; in fact, they are worse because I just want to switch off and relax on a Sunday. In some parts of the Hebrides, even the parks may be closed on Sundays, and although some may feel that this takes the 'day of rest' too far, it is one way of policing the need to keep some time special.

In my experience, many people with chronic pain struggle with the work–life balance, with unofficial work leaking into every aspect of life. Margaret in Blyth told me that she had to prove herself all the time. She said that standards had to be maintained regardless of how she felt and that she never switched off. I asked her, 'Who are you proving yourself to?' Her first reflex was to blame her family, and then her friends, but then the penny dropped and she finally realized that somehow she was trying to prove herself to herself. Sadly, this kind of self-flagellation is very common.

Although many people with chronic pain have had to stop going to work, that does not stop them working – in fact, they often work harder than they ever did before. It is common for people to feel embarrassed, guilty and anxious because they are not working. It is hard to switch off from the need to do jobs to justify one's existence.

Being at home more means that there is often too much time to think too much, with anxiety and unhelpful beliefs brewing up. In this situation, work and worry expand to fill the time available for them. And the increased time to dwell on your life can turn molehills into mountains. This all leads to high levels of stress, pain and fatigue – the very things that you need to avoid, the signs that we are out of balance, or maybe just in the wrong sort of balance.

Work, rest, play

An advert for a certain large bar of chocolate used to say that if you had one it would help you to do your work, to spend time playing and to rest when you needed. These three areas describe a balanced life beautifully. And this is just what Jack needs to do too, balance everything out so it's no longer all work and no play, or even rest for that matter.

However, many people with chronic conditions work too much, only rest when they are exhausted and feel too guilty to enjoy themselves, independently of how many snack bars they eat. Working flat out until you *are* flat out and not having the energy to enjoy life is another example of the boom–bust cycle that was described in Chapter 4 on pacing. It often means that we 'achieve' the opposite of what we need to.

Susan in Dundee had been put on sick leave because of chronic pain and fatigue, but she spent all her time doing housework and actually working harder than when she had been in paid work. Ironically, she was a hospital cleaner, but she cleaned her house more than she had cleaned the hospital. This story has a happy ending though – but I'll keep you in suspense for a while over that.

It is hard to find a balance in life between what we have to do to earn money and keep the home going, and what we like to do to make it all make sense – such as time with family, rest, relaxation, socializing and interests. Many of us are hard on ourselves even when things are going well. And we are often still harder on ourselves if our health changes. Ironically, this is the very time we need to be kinder to ourselves.

Change can create a vacuum, and then guilt and anxiety rush in. This often prompts people to increase their workload at a time in life when they should be adapting to change and doing a bit less. Of course, it is difficult to adapt, especially if you are embarrassed or in denial. The simple outcome is that the work–life balance goes wrong, and people feel worse than they need to. It is vital to find a healthier balance in life.

What I want to ask is: what is *your* work–life balance like? Does it need to change? And if so, what one thing could you do today that would improve the balance? To answer these questions, it helps to see things a little differently.

Fillers and drainers

Hopefully, you are by now realizing that pain is an output from a complex system called You. The important point is that everything that affects you will affect pain or your ability to cope with it. So to improve things, you need to see the big picture.

In the world of health, the humble cup is often used to gain an overview and illustrate ideas that are relevant to maintaining health and well-being. A cup can be half full or half empty, illustrating optimism and pessimism. A cup with a little water can be held at arm's length to show that something which is easy for a short while can become very hard over a prolonged period, as the arm starts to get tired and the glass seems heavier. And if you fill a cup with pebbles representing negatives, there is still lots of room for positives, represented by the sand that can be poured between the pebbles. Giving the 'pebbles' of life a shake-down makes more room for positive 'sand'.

A common non-cup 'cup trick', which people often quote to me as 'the superior one', involves the idea that you have a certain number of spoons and that every time you do something you lose a spoon or two. If you have fewer spoons than you used to have, you need to value your spoons more and think about what you spend them on. I have even met someone who had a spoon necklace to illustrate this. However, I struggle with this a bit because there does not seem to be a way of getting more spoons, which seems rather negative.

My non-cup 'cup trick' is therefore a fuel tank (Figure 10.1). This is all about being aware of your current situation and creating a better balance in life so that you can manage pain better and be happier. It is a kind of 'life audit' to understand and improve health.

Think of your car's fuel tank. You put fuel in, you drive to places, and then when the fuel is running low a light comes on to tell you it is time to fill up. If you ignore the light and keep going, you run out of fuel and get stuck by the roadside. The fuel level is determined by the balance between how much goes in and how much

FILLERS

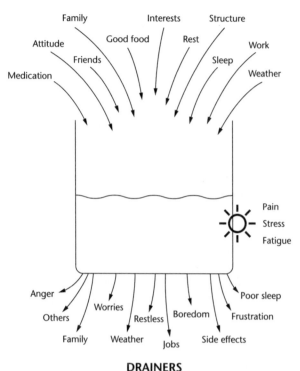

DRAINERS

Figure 10.1 Fillers and drainers

gets used. It makes sense to keep an eye on the fuel level so that you fill up before it is too late.

Some people, like me, always fill up way before the light comes on – my dad told me that if the tank runs low, you dredge up all the sludgy bits at the bottom – but others wait for the alert light to come on, and some even play Russian roulette and see how much they can squeeze out of a tank without grinding to a halt. Interestingly, your relationship with life is a bit like your relationship with your car's fuel tank – so which sort of driver are you?

Although you are not, of course, a car, you work a bit like one. The fuel that we run on is a complex mixture of physical, emotional and social items; I call these fillers. We use our fuel to accomplish tasks that are also physical, emotional, social and environmental, but as they use up fuel, I call these drainers. It would be really useful to have a fuel warning light on your body to keep you notified, but your body finds a way to accomplish that for you. The equivalent of the fuel warning light is the feeling of more pain or fatigue. Other signs of running low are getting stressed, feeling grumpy and feeling claustrophobic. Think of these as the lights and dials on your body's dashboard.

Not surprisingly, people tell me that their pain is usually better when they go on holiday. This is simply because, on holiday, there are more fillers than drainers – assuming of course that it was a stress-free holiday, otherwise the drainers would dominate, the fuel would run low and you would come home with an extra suitcase full of pain, stress and fatigue.

Sarah from Abergele was convinced that it was all about weather. She always went on amazing holidays, and this time she went to New Zealand for a month. She noticed, however, that although the weather was just like that at home (wet!), her pain levels were lower, largely because her holiday was full of fillers compared with life at home.

Try sketching out your own fuel tank as a kind of life audit. You will already have most of it in your mind, but putting it all together and seeing it as a diagram can bring important new insight. Everything is relevant here. Some of the items may explain why you are struggling. Most people seem to have a more draining than filling life. If you have a painful condition, the lower the level in the tank, the more likely you are to have pain.

In one group, we looked at everyone's values and tried to list them in importance. Interestingly, no one had their own health as a value, and everyone had written family at the top of the list. This is common. In fact, people rarely put 'look after myself' as a value. One of the members, Joyce, burst into tears when she drew her fuel tank, because she realized that her needy mother-in-law was an enormous drain on her. Joyce's story was a positive one because once she realized what was happening, when she literally saw it in black and white, it motivated her to do something about it.

Joyce, like other group members, had put family at the top of her list, but when she looked at her diagram, she realized that her mother-in-law was draining her excessively, so much so that it was using all her energy. This meant that Joyce had nothing left for her husband and children. Once she realized this, she had a chat with her mother-in-law to limit the drainers. Joyce explained that when she visited, she could only stay for an hour at a time, and that she would not always be able to come round when she was called. In addition, when her mother-in-law rang, she would have to limit the time on the phone. Joyce recognized that her mother-in-law had needs, and she wanted to support her, but she also realized that she could not afford to be so seriously drained.

Earlier in the chapter I mentioned Susan who, despite being on sick leave, was working harder at home than she did at work. When she drew her own fuel tank, she saw that it was non-stop drain and no fill. She decided that she needed two hours of downtime every day. During this downtime, she just did whatever she felt like doing – from watching TV to visiting a friend. The result was that she got back to work sooner than she might have. Put simply, every day she added two hours of fuel into her tank, and by addressing her deficit in this way, she put herself back in balance.

Finding the right balance in life is vital for health. And if your health has changed, it is critical to rebalance life. This will involve making changes and new choices.

Balance the Chinese way

It seems odd, but everything in life always tries to find a balance. At a simple level, if you feel hungry you eat, if you are tired you sleep, if you are hot you sweat to cool down, and if you are cold you shiver to warm up. If you injure yourself, you feel pain and that forces you to protect the damaged area until it heals. All of this is the body putting you in balance with your environment – the process of balancing the systems within the body is called homeostasis, which simply means physiological stability.

If you are doing too much and feeling dreadful, the balance you are in is an unpleasant one. Just like when we are hot or cold, this feeling should, in theory, prompt us to take action to set up a better balance. However, it is easy to ignore how we feel, thinking that it is just a medical issue that we cannot affect, and soldiering on.

The idea of balance is ancient. It's even older than Jack in his seventeenth-century field. It is the basis for several significant holistic approaches to health. One of the oldest is traditional Chinese medicine, whose main objective is to focus on finding a good balance. European physicians in the Middle Ages were also doing something similar when they looked to balance the 'five humours'. In traditional Chinese medicine, everything is about finding balance, and this is often illustrated by the familiar symbol that shows two aspects of life: Yin and Yang.

Put too simply, Yin is cool, night, light, winter, rest and female, while Yang is hot, day, summer, active and male. A lovely balanced meal for instance often has meat (Yang) and vegetables (Yin). Both are necessary for there to be a balance. Some people have Yang constitutions and are prone to 'hot' conditions such as inflammation; others are Yin by nature and develop conditions such as fatigue. We are all one or the other, and this means we all need different things to obtain a good balance. Yang people need to go on holiday in Iceland, while Yin folk need the sun in Benidorm. A clue to your Yinness or Yangness is to realize what weather makes you feel best. One of the most famous lines in Chinese medicine is: 'If Yin and Yang are balanced in form, our essence and spirit will be good.'

This basically means that balance is central to everything, and hopefully I've made that point too.

Change and choice

As I said in relation to pacing in Chapter 4, Chinese philosopher Lao Tzu once wisely wrote, 'If you do not change direction, you may end up where you are heading'. A change in health often means that we have much less fuel than we used to, but the temptation is to carry on regardless. This means we will keep running out of fuel. It usually takes a while for us to realize this, but in the end we need to make some choices about how we use our precious but limited fuel. It's the old story of needing to budget better or 'cut your coat according to your cloth'.

Thinking of this in terms of the fuel tank, it is helpful to assess the relative merits of the things you use your fuel on. If nothing changes, you will keep running out of fuel. This exercise is a classic cost–benefit analysis but can be simplified to just asking yourself the following: Is it worth it? Do I have to? Can I afford it?

Assessing the relative worth of what you do is up to you. It is not all about avoiding pain because sometimes what you do is worth the pain you might cause. The key is to understand your body and to exercise a choice. It's a bit like, as we saw in Chapter 4, a hangover – someone might say never again after having too much to drink, but when the next day comes, they are back in the pub for the next knees up.

The whole concept of 'choice' can be difficult because some people believe that they genuinely do not have any. This may just be because they are not used to the idea. Obviously there are some things, such as going to the toilet or crossing the road, where choice is limited, but there are always some issues in life, even just small ones, where it is possible to make a different choice.

Many years ago, I did a job I totally disliked. Then someone who could see how fed up I was remarked, 'You do know you have a choice, don't you?' I growled a bit and rejected the statement for a while, but I realized that I felt I did not have a choice simply because I was too scared and did not have the confidence to leave the job. Realizing this then helped me to find a new post. So if you feel that you do not have a choice, I can empathize, but remember that we sometimes choose not to have a choice because it is more comfortable to stick with the familiar or just too hard to think of an alternative.

Even a small change to a minor aspect of life will get the choice ball rolling: 'The journey of a thousand miles starts with one step', as Lao Tzu also wisely said. Make a few small choices about your fillers and drainers – ideally to achieve greater filling while also doing something to reduce the draining. You do not have to jettison something completely, just to do it differently so that it is less draining.

Summary

If the balance of life has changed, we need to change with it or something will give. In the case of chronic pain, this will produce greater pain and a worse feeling. It is easy to get stuck, but if you can start to see things in a different way, to recognize your fillers and drainers, it will give you a new way of thinking about the world that will help you to find a new balance and change your world.

'Better the devil you know' creates a lot of misery. It is a kind of comfortably uncomfortable. It's good to change it because there might be an angel round the corner.

Part 3
COPING

11

The principles of coping

Problems are not the problem; coping is the problem.

Virginia Satir

It goes without saying, but I will say it anyway – chronic pain is hard to cope with. It catches everyone out. We're not prepared for it, we don't expect it, it's hard to make sense of, it follows you around all day, it seems unfair, it's stressful, you can't see it, few understand what you are going through, there are no easy answers and it's difficult to accept. If you wanted to make something really hard to cope with, this would be how to do it!

That is not to say, of course, that your condition is the only challenge you are trying to cope with. Everyone has many other life challenges, such as stress at work or relationship issues, but a change in health means that most people have far more on their plate than they used to. In Chapter 1, I referred to this as having a bigger knot. To add metaphors, this extra length of spaghetti on your plate, this extra strand in your knot, can be the straw that breaks the camel's back. Put simply, people are often overloaded and live on the limit, so it is easy to become overwhelmed.

We all cope in our own way. Some ways such as rationalizing, relaxing and making sure you have support are helpful. Others aren't – self-harm, drinking and isolating yourself fall into this category. But however ugly and destructive the action is, it still represents an attempt to cope. Whatever you do to cope, the instinct is the same: to quieten the mind, seek comfort and get through things without falling apart. And there is usually room for improvement in our strategies.

The scope of coping

I see pain management as lightening the load. This simply means helping people to cope better with their burdens. Some things are directly related to pain, but many indirect issues add to the load. Whether or not the pain is changing, it is important to look at every aspect of your life and improve whatever you can.

If you have made your load lighter, if you have changed what you can change, then there is more capacity for coping with what you cannot change right now. It's like being a weight-lifter: if you have less to lift, you will lift it more easily.

Two-stage coping – the tyranny of housework

As mentioned above, there are obvious good and bad approaches to coping, but there is a third category. This is where some parts of the approach are helpful but after a while it backfires.

An example of this two-stage coping is housework. This is a good choice because a lot of people say they're a 'bit OCD about it'. This phrase itself rings alarm bells. Housework is a big hook that people get caught on, and it is often at the centre of discussions about adapting to change. I have lost count of the number of discussions I have had about housework over the years. Happily, I have helped to make the world slightly less tidy.

On the face of it, housework can seem a good way to cope. It ticks lots of boxes but, crucially, only to a point. The potential advantages are that it is distracting, it is a way to feel in control, it is something to be proud of, it is a response to deal with some of the guilt, it gives a sense of purpose and it involves acting on familiar rules and certainties.

The trouble is that it is easy to get carried away. Housework is a hard taskmaster because it is a fast track to feeling bad if you don't do it like your mum did. But, most importantly, it never finishes. So what starts out as a good way to channel your energies ends up using them all up. In many ways, it is a wolf in sheep's clothing – and you'd have to vacuum a lot if you had both of them in the house!

The 3 Rs

Coping is an odd thing because we are doing it all the time, but we rarely step back and think about what we are actually doing. We probably picked up our coping style from our parents and revert to it in difficult times without reviewing whether or not it is helping. It seems to be an unconscious reflex, which means we can be surprised by our reactions in different situations. Like everything unconscious, it is helpful to have a look at coping and see what we are supposed to do, see how we measure up and whether we can identify anything we could do better.

Coping well involves the '3 Rs':

- reducing the difficulty itself (practical problem-solving);
- responding helpfully (attitude and emotions);
- research (finding out in a way that helps with the first two points).

As a simple example, imagine your neighbour was playing loud music. Using the 3 Rs, you could:

- R1: Tell them to turn it down or cut the mains cable (a practical approach).
- R2: See it from the perspective of 'I want to be a tolerant neighbour', 'Maybe they don't realize how loud their music is', 'We had a party last week that they didn't complain about' or 'I'll give it a bit but then I'll have to say something' (responding).
- R3: Find out why they are playing the music. Maybe it is just for a short time or perhaps there is a children's party (research).

Let's apply this to the more serious situation of a flare-up.

- R1: You may struggle to reduce the pain itself, but you can address wider issues – cancel commitments that you are not up to meeting, cut back on the usual jobs and make sure you get more rest (practical).
- R2: Remind yourself that the situation will pass, and that your low mood is due to the pain (responding). Focus on staying calm and rationalizing your thoughts (responding).
- R3: You know how long it will last (research), and you can use this to reassure yourself that it usually settles after a few days (responding).

This list of 3 Rs is not exhaustive – it is just a good way to remember the key ingredients of coping – and you may like to add your own points. Another memorable acronym for the same topics is PEA (Practical, Emotional, Ask).

The key to coping well is to use a mix of these approaches – one approach on its own does not sort everything. In addition, most people have a 'go to' approach that is based on what they are good at. I will probably get into trouble for saying this, but men and women also tend to cope differently. Men often seek a practical approach, whereas women prefer to talk about the emotions involved. These are, however, just broad generalizations, and you are allowed to be different from the stereotype!

Understanding your main coping strength is helpful because you can work out what you need help with. Similarly, understanding another's coping strength can be useful if they want to help you. For example, if you have a partner who is a practical person, asking them to understand how you feel is futile. Give them something to do though, and they will be happy. It is important to recognize that accepting help helps others to cope too. It gives them something to put their 'care energy' into.

Techniques

Modelling

There is a tradition in positive approaches to health in which you look at what successful people do and then you copy them. This kind of modelling makes a great deal of sense. If someone has already gone there and got the experience, let that help you. If that is a friend, you are even more likely to respect what they have done and apply it to yourself. This works really well in group work, where people learn from others in a similar situation and can see that there is light at the end of the tunnel.

Coping with pain is no different in principle from any kind of coping in difficult circumstances because it is all about life. Think for instance about how people you know have coped with major stressors such as bereavement, redundancy or divorce. Most importantly, think about how you have coped in the past with your own troubles. What have you learnt about how you cope? What is your main coping strength? What helps you? What doesn't? What do you need to add?

Modelling yourself on others who have faced similar situations is gold dust. However, we also need to give ourselves credit for what we have done well in the past and remind ourselves that we can still do it. In this way, you are then modelling yourself on the capable you.

Coping well involves the mix of skills that were summarized above as the 3 Rs. The greater detail of coping involves: the right attitude, problem-solving, realism, communication, putting things in context, information, staying calm, getting help, humour, being proportionate, acceptance, and belief in yourself. This could read like an impossible shopping list, but you might surprise yourself when you consider what you have been able to do in the past.

Living with pain erodes confidence and self-esteem, and we often think that we are failing when we are actually doing rather well. In fact, living with chronic pain takes a great deal of courage and energy all on its own. Giving yourself credit for coping is a way to improve that coping, and this will spur you on to see yourself in a more positive light.

Below are a few extra tools and ideas that are worth adding to the coping toolbox.

The magic wand

Magic wand thinking is really useful in problem-solving. It would obviously be better to have a real wand, like Harry Potter's, but we will have to make do with imagining one instead. What then would be the magic solution you would conjure up? This slightly silly exercise somehow helps you to realize what the priority is.

Anne had been talking to me about how a tidy house helped her to cope with pain. But making the house perfect made her pain worse. When we 'used' the magic wand, her wish was, not surprisingly, for less pain. So I asked her how the magic wand could get that for her. And then the penny dropped that she needed to do less of the housework that was causing it. As a result, she cut her housework burden down by enlisting her daughter's help.

The magic wand's solution will often be one that is not immediately possible right now but it will indicate the right direction. Tom's magic wand answer was 'Win the lottery' – an obviously tricky proposition – but this idea was the trigger for him to seek financial advice about how to deal with his debts.

Can versus can't

It's easy to focus on what you *can't* do. This is a stage in the acceptance process that we will look at later, but for now it is important to focus on the practical idea: if you focus on what you cannot do, it will block you from doing what you can do. So the big question is, what can I do now? This is often helped by reducing the scale and time of the response to, what one thing could I do *now*, no matter how small, that would make a difference? Making a difference could be one of the 3 Rs or PEA items, that is, practical, emotional or finding out.

Prioritizing

With limited resources, it is hard to do everything you used to. Prioritizing means that you will do what is most important first. It also means that you can plan to achieve what you most need to based on your values. This is critically important in maximizing choice, which is decided on by the process of weighing up cost versus benefit.

Better out than in

My dad often said this about flatulence! But in fact it's true for most things. It is much better to talk about something that is bothering you than to hold it all in. Talking helps to put things in context and might lead you to the solution – this is basically what happens in counselling. It also helps to express and let go of your emotions. If, for instance, you are angry, it is better to punch a punchbag than yourself or someone else. Many people benefit from expressing their feelings through art. One lady who attended one of my pain management courses showed me her 'before' and 'after' pictures – the pre-course pictures were full of black, block-like shapes, whereas the post-course picture was lighter and brighter.

On this theme, some researchers from Keele University found that swearing helped people who had pain. I'm not suggesting you go around swearing at the world, but again, better out than in.

Keep calm

I cannot overstate the importance of being calmer. Quite simply, when we are calmer, we are less emotional and more rational. The angry, stressed person will not be able to see beyond their 'red mist', but when they are calmer the world is a better place and the wood emerges from the trees. This is why it is crucial to step back and remember to 'cool your jets'.

The classic advice to stop and take a few slow breaths is incredibly useful. This may be hard when you are raging with emotion, but it is the very thing that you need to do to cope better. Make sure you adopt the techniques outlined in Chapter 6 on relaxation, especially those on breathing and anchoring.

Break outdated patterns

You may remember, in Chapter 4 on pacing, the repeating T-shirt slogan 'Frustration, Pain, Collapse, Repeat'. This can become a self-fulfilling prophesy that keeps running like a computer program. This is why it is important to break the pattern of life. Think of it as rebooting the computer program that you are living. This sounds a bit like being in the film *The Matrix*, but try it.

Start with driving home a different way, or watching something new on TV. These may be small steps, but they get your unconscious mind thinking that things can be different. A colleague who is very keen on this approach says he gets dressed in a different way every day, maybe right sock, left sleeve, right leg, with odd episodes of falling over. The point is an important one – it's easy to get stuck in a groove that keeps repeating itself like Groundhog Day.

Find meaning

It is crucial to have large projects and passions that give life meaning and focus. This is especially important when life has become limited and the focus has turned to pain and its conse-quences. It is also crucial not to let pain take everything away.

One lady I worked with was an artist. She said that she was going to give up painting because it increased her pain. I explained to her that it was vital she kept painting because, if she gave that up, she would have nothing positive to focus on. Going deeper, it would undoubtedly make her pain worse because it would increase her sadness – it would mean that she was no longer an artist. Maintaining – or taking up – new hobbies and interests is vital to keep life interesting, generate things to look forward to and give us a sense of achievement and pride.

When to ignore yourself

When we are facing difficulties, when we are stressed and struggling to cope, an unwelcome visitor often pops up. This is a particular kind of unhelpful thought that people in the world of CBT call a 'NAT' (negative automatic thought), but I prefer to call it a NAG (negative automatic garbage) because that is how it feels. A NAG is a rubbishy old belief that undermines confidence. It is like having the opposite of a supportive personal trainer – with a NAG, you have someone who is shouting your weaknesses and insecurities at you.

The NAG might remind you of your worst fears, or your sensitivities, or your lifelong emotional baggage. The key point is that these are usually entirely out of date and no longer relevant. It is important to spot this and know that you need to resist the pull. There are some classics here.

- 'You're no good.'
- 'You should do better.'
- 'You don't belong.'
- 'The worst always happens.'
- 'Your best isn't good enough.'

If someone else said these unpleasant things to you, you would be very upset and tell them they were wrong. But somehow, if you say them to yourself, you listen carefully and take it all in, lock, stock and barrel.

NAGs are challenged in therapy by asking about their relevance and any evidence for them being correct. The key here is to be aware of them and to realize that they come out to play when you are under pressure. Sometimes we are stuck with a NAG for life. Maybe a leopard cannot change its spots, but you can certainly make them less sticky. We need to see NAGs for what they are: old rubbish that no longer belongs with you. If you spot them, blow them a raspberry and carry on regardless.

Behave like you are coping

Arriving on time and keeping up personal standards in dress and appearance are very important because they are things you can do, they communicate things about you to the world around, and this feeds back to you in a positive way. As the saying goes, you get back what you give out. Feeling that others think positively about you is an important part of coping.

See beyond the situation

Focusing on something difficult or new, such as an appointment, a job interview or even a pain management course, can be worrying. This can lead us to prepare for it in an unhelpful way. You can, however, bounce in full of a far more helpful set of thoughts if you focus on thinking about what it will be like after the event. For instance, I hate DIY with a passion, largely because I have no clue about what I'm doing, so I have to focus on thinking about what it will be like when I've finished – about how it good it will look, and how nice it will be to have that glass of wine as a reward. This is a simple example but it gives the idea of how focusing beyond a challenge lifts the spirits and enables you to get through it in good form.

Fillers and drainers

Going back to the balance of life that I discussed in the fuel tank example in Chapter 10, if you have got more fuel in the tank, everything is easier to cope with because you have the resources (the fuel) that you need. Coping better means that less fuel gets burnt too, but remembering to keep the tank's level up is critical for coping in the first place.

Coping versus pain

Alison in Hexham was a bit puzzled. She said that she had had guests for a few months and that she had got out of her usual pain management routine. She wanted to get that routine back, but when we spoke she said that her pain had been worse but she had coped better than normal. We discussed how having things to look forward to, enjoying life and improving her mood were all helping her to cope better. Rather than resurrect all her old ways, she needed to stick with the things that had improved her ability to cope. It showed that focusing on coping was more important than worrying about pain levels.

Summary

Coping is a mix of problem-solving, calmness and attitude. Some people are natural copers, but like everything this is something that you can learn to do better. In many ways, how well you cope is more important than what you're coping with.

12

Acceptance

What we resist persists.

Carl Jung

Whenever I mention acceptance, there is often a sharp intake of breath. Like 'pacing', it is one of those 'Marmite' words.

The crossed arms and glaring expressions I encounter are based on a misunderstanding about what acceptance really means. Some people think it means giving up and giving in, but it is really about coming to terms with change so that it no longer runs your life. Acceptance means being able to look at something square in the face and do something about it. The proper sense of acceptance is that you see difficulties and changes for what they are, stop trying to ignore them and get on with life. But I know that this is easy to say and hard to do.

Change

The process of coming to terms with any major change is hard for most people. Redundancy, divorce and bereavement all take a lot of adjusting to. People often say that life is just not the same any more, and some may never get over the event.

Similarly, a change in health is a major shock that is tough to deal with. It may be especially hard because chronic pain is not something that many people are familiar with. It also tends to interfere with many aspects of life and reminds you unpleasantly (through its symptoms) of its presence. In addition, the variable nature of pain means that the situation varies from day to day; during a flare-up, for example, acceptance goes backwards for a while.

In pain management, it is vital to move from fighting against your condition to managing it. To make this move, it is necessary to understand more about your situation, untangle facts from emotional responses, think about your priorities and maybe redefine what you expect and hope for. It sounds cheesy to say it, but it's a journey.

Stages of bereavement model

The classical Kübler-Ross model of bereavement is very helpful when thinking about the journey to acceptance. It is otherwise known as the five stages of grief model. It says that, when someone dies, we go through a process of adjusting to the change that is characterized by different emotional stages. This model can also be used to help understand other major changes, such as a change in health. The stages are listed below and can be remembered by its letters as DABDA. I've added my own comments to make them relevant to chronic pain.

- **Denial** 'That can't have happened, I'll just carry on regardless.'
- **Anger** 'Why me? The doctors are useless.'
- **Bargaining** 'I'll try and look after my health better, if only the pain will go away.'
- **Depression** 'I feel down, I give up, I'm on the scrapheap, I've no choice.'
- **Acceptance** 'Things are as they are. I need to manage and cope, and get on with life.'

We go through a version of these stages even for the minor situations in life. Think of breaking down in your brand new Rolls Royce car:

- **Denial** 'Rolls-Royces *never* break down.'
- **Anger** 'I must have been sold a dud. Why me?'
- **Bargaining** 'If I stay stuck, I won't get home so I'll need to do something.'
- **Depression** 'I give up.'
- **Acceptance** 'I'll ring my breakdown service.'

The stages

The idea is that we go through these stages over time. Several stages might happen at the same time, and you can go backwards and forwards through them, or repeat them. To customize the situation of chronic pain in a health setting, we could add other pertinent emotions, such as guilt, frustration and bewilderment. People are generally never happy that something bad has happened, but they learn to live with it. Many people have told me that they continue to feel the emotions, but they get easier with time. So the first encouragement I can offer is that the situation will usually improve with time.

This emotional process of going through the stages is natural and a necessary part of adjusting to change. If someone jumps straight to acceptance, the emotions often hit them later. This is particularly the case with people who have experienced traumatic events, held it all in and appeared to cope – and then it hits them hard later on. It can also hit them hard in a different way because emotions that are held in often get expressed in a different form later, and this can include pain.

It helps to be able to identify the stage you are at. It helps to explain why you are reacting to the world as you are. With time, and with dealing with it, that stage will improve and then pass. The key is not to get stuck for too long. I know a few people who have become stuck at the anger stage; this now runs their lives and winds the pain up at every turn.

What helps?

It helps to be able to express emotions and act on them when appropriate, to find out information about your condition, to meet others in a similar situation, to reduce stress and to understand that the way you see the world right now might be because you are going through a process of change. This is especially important because someone in the early stages of the process will struggle to see how the future could possibly turn out positively.

Hope helps. Many people talk about feeling helpless and hopeless. That is no surprise because if you do not think anything will help your situation, if you think you are stuck with it, then it makes sense to feel hopeless. This is where you need a positive experience, anything that will turn a light on at the end of the tunnel. I often find that people who learn to relax suddenly see the future differently. I have also seen someone in a group provide hope to another by saying, 'I was like you when I came, but things improved for me.'

It is easy to feel hopeless. A man came to a group once, but he didn't even stay long enough for me to find out his name. He turned up late and looked miserable. He clearly didn't want to be with me. When he spoke, he dismissed what I was saying with 'The surgeon said I'd only get worse.' I'm sure that's not all the surgeon said, but that's what he had come away with.

What I wanted to do was to get him to see things from a different perspective. I wanted to say: when you understand pain, you will realize that changes in the body do not necessarily equate to changes in pain. I wanted to say that even if his condition did get worse, he could get stronger in himself, learn some techniques, reduce stress, feel supported and have more in his life than his condition. I wanted to say all these things, but he was out of the room in flash. He was at a stage that was overwhelming him, creating a black view of the future and blocking out any messages of hope.

Overaccepting

Just to make things tricky, overaccepting can also cause difficulties. In this situation, someone can define themselves by their condition. The thinking tends to be mostly passive and couched in terms of what *cannot* be done, such as, 'With my condition, you can't sleep'. This tends to be the sort of 'surrender' that most people would be wary of. The best balance lies somewhere between not liking what has happened but being in a position to do something positive about it.

One lady I met who had been talking in Internet chat rooms for fibromyalgia for too long announced: 'I've decided I am my condition'. I tried to suggest that she was herself first and her condition second, but she was not keen on that idea. Maybe it was part of her acceptance journey, or maybe it was just her way of coping for that time in her life.

Time frame

Acceptance is hard, especially when we see the rest of life as an inevitable decline. Niall in Dublin said he could not accept anything, and that if he paced himself, this would mean that he accepted his condition. I suggested that he focus on pacing his activities as a purely practical exercise to help with his pain, and to try to forget all the 'big stuff' for now. The trouble was that Niall's fear of acceptance was stopping him from doing something that would make his situation a little easier, and ironically make it easier to accept. He needed to just *do it*. Niall seemed both surprised and relieved at this, and then started to say that he might change in time. So suddenly he was more positive when he thought he was off the acceptance hook.

Acceptance of everything is often too hard, especially when we see it from a difficult place where there is currently no sense of hope. It is also hard when someone else tells you that you have to accept it. You know that, but doing it is a different matter. Try focusing on what you can accept right now, realizing that you can accept in stages, like paying for a sofa in instalments. For example, as you are reading this book, you are doing something to move along the acceptance curve. This may sound trivial, but it is important to point out any successes you have with acceptance.

Summary

If you focus on doing what you *can* do rather than what you *can't*, if you do something differently, like Niall did, the future changes. Acceptance is easier when hope is rekindled. If we resist something and do nothing about it, if we try to look the other way, nothing changes.

I always suggest that people forget accepting for now and start adapting.

13

Kindness

No act of kindness, no matter how small, is ever wasted.

Aesop

If you boil pain management down to its absolute essence, it is simply all about being kinder to yourself. It might sound disappointing that it's not a cutting-edge technology or an ancient Buddhist technique, or maybe it is, but it is probably the oldest idea going. The reason that kindness is so important is that most people give themselves a hard time when their health changes. In fact, most people give themselves a hard time all the time regardless.

When change occurs, it unsettles us and seems to draw in lots of stress, anxiety and self-doubt; in short, change sucks in all sorts of rubbish. If you cannot do what you used to do, it is easy to feel bad, feel ashamed and try to keep things the same – this means that we keep pushing hard when the body is screaming STOP. I'm not saying that you should not try hard – in fact you are probably trying harder than everyone else – but you should do this within limits. With chronic pain, there is far more than 'just pain' going on. Lots of additional suffering comes from being hard on yourself and not allowing yourself to adapt to change.

Ironically, most people say that being kind is one of their most important values. Many would say that they put their needs last and are kind to everyone except themselves. The cheeky questions to ask are: 'If you value kindness so much, why don't you apply it to yourself?' 'Why treat yourself worse than others?' 'Why do for others what you won't do for yourself?' 'Why tell others to do the things you don't do yourself?' One answer is that it is easy to be kind to others, whereas being kind to yourself runs headlong into issues of self-esteem and other emotional baggage.

It's a great quality to be kind, so please don't stop – but the point I want to make is to be kinder to yourself. This is not just a twee idea, but a practical one, and it will help you to be more reliably kind. If you follow it through it can be an incredibly powerful philosophy that unhooks you from all sorts of misery.

The *Oxford English Dictionary* defines kindness as 'the quality of being friendly, generous and considerate'. This is about caring, valuing and seeing people as people. It means accepting people for who they are and maybe forgiving them from time to time. In short, it is a form of practical love. If you give it out all the time, you might not be aware of what exactly it would be like to be kind to yourself. My suggestion is that it would mean:

- forgiving yourself – it's fine not to be fine;
- being generous – to yourself;
- valuing yourself;
- not always putting your own needs last;
- not being so hard on yourself;
- giving yourself permission to look after yourself;
- respecting your own values and needs;
- not needing to seek permission from others, but doing what you know will be good for you;
- not needing to justify yourself through non-stop work;
- not feeling guilty if you are enjoying yourself;
- less 'ought, should and must';
- less self-critical thinking;
- knowing it's fine just to be yourself;
- recognizing your achievements and efforts;
- allowing compliments in;
- dismissing unwarranted criticism;
- judging yourself by effort and not achievement;
- accepting help.

Reading through this list might make you squirm, but it is probably what you urge others to do. All I am doing is suggesting that you consider aiming some of it at yourself, so that you occasionally put your needs first, you look after yourself more, and you do not beat yourself up so much with guilt or worry about what others think.

Of course, you might say 'yes, but . . .':

- 'I've no choice';
- 'I can't change';

- 'people expect me to do everything.'

Lower your defences for a while and let a bit of kindness in. This makes sense for several reasons:

- because you are worth it;
- because others want you to;
- because if you don't, you won't be able to do what is important to you – probably being kind to others.

The first of these does not usually convince anyone, but the second and third do. It is a simple case of logic – if you do not look after yourself, you will not be able to do the things that are most important to you. And when I ask people what is most important to them, the top three are:

- being kind;
- caring for family;
- being there for people.

Accepting help

There are two sources of kindness: other people and yourself. Sometimes you might block kindnesses from others because you want to do it all yourself, you want to be independent and you want to do it to your own high standard. But what if all that blocking is making you worse? You might also be complaining that 'no one helps, no one cares, no one understands', when in fact you might be blocking other people from helping you, not because you do not want help, but because pride, embarrassment and independence are getting in the way. An important issue in accepting help is that we are not used to people being nice to us.

You might worry unnecessarily about what it would be like, and maybe worry that your standards would go to pot – although I am sure that the standards argument is usually used as an excuse to prevent embarrassment or a feeling of being looked down on. But those who want to help are desperate to see you have an easier time. They want to help for the right reasons. Remember though that if you don't care about yourself, it will feel wrong that someone is trying to care for you.

Practical kindness

Thinking about some of the points from the previous pages, I would like you to ask yourself the following questions in just the same caring way that you would ask them of a friend: What am I trying to achieve? Is it realistic? Is it worth it? Is there a better way? What needs to change? And most importantly: What about me? This all looks a bit like needing to be assertive – but in fact it relates more to being clear about your values. At this stage, it might be worth stepping back and giving yourself a little time to reflect on what is most important to you, that is, what exactly your values are.

What is most important to you? You may remember Joyce in Chapter 10 on balance, who had to think about how much energy she was using up on caring for her mother-in-law. She found that family was her most important value, but to deliver on that value she needed to keep a bit of fuel in the tank for herself to maintain her health. The kindness she showed to herself was a practical kindness that achieved something important. It did not beg awkward questions about self-esteem; rather it was just about being honest with herself.

Forced kindness

We sometimes behave 'kindly' not because we really want to, but because we feel that we do not have a choice. If we appear kind to everyone else, is that really because we are kind or because we are stuck in a certain role and cannot say no?

Summary

Kindness is not just a twee hippy idea, it is a practical issue. Being kinder to yourself is nothing to do with lazing about eating choco-lates and saying 'I'm worth it'. Instead, it is about being realistic about your needs and values and letting yourself do things in a way that achieves them. It is also about accepting help and letting nice people in.

Kindness needs to go in all directions, to others and to you.

14

Reframing – daring to be positive

We're all in the gutter, but some of us are looking at the stars.

Oscar Wilde

It sounds obvious, but it's worth saying anyway: the way we see the world is the way we get the world. And what we 'see' varies widely. Some see good things, others only difficulties. The difference lies in how we think about ourselves and the context that we use to interpret events. A good way of describing the 'context' is as the 'frame' that we put around things.

This does not stop with thinking as thinking affects behaviour and stirs up emotions. This is all very important because people often construct frames that cause many problems. If, for instance, you think of yourself as a failure, you will often interpret events as confirming to you that you are a failure. This can easily lead to negative experiences that include low mood, sensitivity to others' comments and withdrawal from important activities.

As I said above, the way we see the world is the way we get the world. If you are getting the world in an unpleasant way, it is important to try to change the way that you see it. In short, change your thinking and you will change your world.

Here is another way of putting this: the way we think about the world creates behaviours, mood and actions, so changing our thinking can improve our mood, behaviours and actions. This is of course easy to say, but possibly hard to imagine working. A more radical way of looking at this is to just start behaving more positively and our thinking and mood will join in. It's the basis of 'fake it to make it'.

It is always important to be realistic, so I am not expecting you to turn mud into gold in an instant. Instead, you need to chip away at your views to change the way you interpret the world. But remember that even trying is a good start.

Reframing your thoughts

Deliberately changing the way you choose to think about things is generally known as 'reframing'. This is the equivalent of replacing a cheap picture frame with a smarter one. Having a posh frame means that we might at least consider that the picture is good, or just expensive, and therefore we will value it more. Sometimes the right frame brings out things in the picture that you never noticed before.

Reframing is not a new concept. We often talk about 'seeing the world through rose-tinted glasses' when someone is being unrealistically positive. We also commonly say 'worse things happen at sea', 'every cloud has a silver lining' and 'always look on the bright side of life'. Reframing is the deliberate use of a positive point of view. It is important in enabling us to cope with difficulties and put aside feelings that might otherwise make a difficult situation worse. It is a simple way of focusing on the positive rather than the negative aspects of a situation.

In my experience, there are two extremely powerful examples of reframing that are central to improving coping strategies:

- 'What I don't have' is reframed into 'What I do have'.
- 'What I can't do' is reframed into 'What I can do'.

Try thinking in these terms when you are feeling anxious or overwhelmed by a situation. Simply changing the way you talk to yourself at least forces you to consider the possibility that there are positive as well as negative ways of seeing the same situation. Unfortunately, seeing things in a negative context often seems easier than seeing them in a positive context, especially if we are not used to doing this or we feel that we do not have permission to reframe things. Put simply, familiar unpleasant frames are easier to have than lovely new ones, but that doesn't mean that you can't do it. Here are some further examples that you can try.

- Change, 'I only did half the job' to, 'I've got the job half done.'
- Change, 'I'm a failure' to, 'Things have changed. I do my best.'
- Change, 'I can't do it like I used to' to, 'I've found a new way to do it.'
- Change, 'What if the worst happens?' to, 'What if the best happens?' or 'What if nothing happens?'
- Change, 'The glass is half empty' to, 'The glass is half full.'

Uses and abuses

We have a deep-rooted cultural suspicion of using positive rather than negative language. Negative thinking tends to be easier than positive thinking. What is wrong will usually overwhelm what is right. And complaining is more common than praising.

There are plenty examples of 'reframing' being used to deceive us, such as estate agents describing a house with no walls as being 'well ventilated', or politicians avoiding the question by focusing on what they have done rather than on what they have failed to do. Luckily, we can see through these as cynical attempts to distort things to the speaker's advantage. This is reframing in negative hands.

In your hands, however, reframing could help you to at least consider an alternative version of events – that there is good even when you may think everything is overwhelmingly bad. You will also have the discernment to know if you are conning yourself.

What's your frame?

Whenever a person considers anything, they start imposing their 'frame' on it. Try this. Try doing anything without interpreting it, thinking about whether it is good or not, predicting what might go wrong or right, and so on. It is always hard to see things for what they are rather than what we think they are.

There are as many versions of an event as there are people experiencing it. There is no need to worry if your version of events works for you, but if it does it is still important to reflect on the 'frame' that you are using. Even if you cannot be positive, maybe try being less negative, even a little bit, however hard it is. That little 'bit' might be sufficient to free you from unhelpful moods and behaviours that could be perpetuating a difficult situation.

Choice

It is odd, but also liberating, to think that we do not have to think what we have always thought, that we might be wrong and that there might be an alternative version of events. In short, we have a choice in the way we think. We do not have to think the way that we do – we might just have got into the habit over years of practice. Virtually everyone falls into the habit of interpreting the world in a certain way. This can be so strong that contemplating an alternative will seem impossible and irrational, when in fact it may just be unfamiliar.

Overcoming reluctance

As a motivation to overcome a reluctance to try reframing, consider that negative framing is just as prejudiced and 'inaccurate' as positive framing. So you might as well be 'wrong' and happy as 'wrong' and miserable.

Reframing properly applied is a way of helping you to escape from a thinking trap 'frame' that might have made a difficult situation harder for a long time. It is therefore worth making a major effort to overcome your reservations and give it a try. It might change things a small amount or a lot, but it can only improve things. To reframe this latter possibility, try entertaining the idea that 'it might work' rather than 'it won't work'.

Breaking the habits of old thinking and trying out a different version of things (an alternative frame) allows you to try out a new construction of the world. At first, this will seem odd and uncomfortable, but with time the new approach will bring benefits and you might even surprise yourself.

How to do it

Use reframing in a way that works for you. Most people simply say something to themselves, usually silently but also out loud if no one else can hear. Others write a key phrase on a bit of paper. Others might get friends or family involved in reminding them to reframe when things are getting difficult. Physical reminders (objects, jewellery, a knotted handkerchief) can act as aids and can be part of a useful habit; for example, when you look at your watch, remind yourself to think positively.

Reframing works best if you keep trying. At first, you might feel awkward and resist what you are saying to yourself. But keep trying, adjust your message to suit you and eventually you could end up just thinking more positively without having to remind yourself.

When to do it

Try reframing in different situations:

- when you are getting anxious about something;
- when you are getting wound up during an event;
- after the event when you might be turning things over and over in your head;
- any time you catch yourself feeling low, angry, frustrated or anxious.

Self-awareness

Looking at a self-awareness habit is also a good exercise for everyone to do from time to time. Ask yourself, 'How am I seeing the world at the moment? What's on my mind? What is colouring my thinking? Is it realistic? Am I thinking too much? Am I too sensitive about a particular issue?' It may be useful to ask others to comment on how they think you might be seeing the world.

Positivity – it's infectious

If you are trying to be more positive yourself, other people will start to warm to this. This is not saying laugh when you want to cry, but instead make a general effort to be positive; this will often improve relationships with family and friends. And this situation in turn may help you to stay more positive.

Summary

It is difficult to be positive and easy to be negative, especially when things have changed and life is harder than it used to be. Reframing gives a simple but effective way to begin to move forward. It will not solve everything, but with practice it will start to sink in and could help create an important improvement. It is not a magic trick, but making an effort to see things in a different context is important if you are not currently doing this.

Most clouds have a silver lining, it just depends how we look at them. Sometimes this takes effort, but it's worth it.

15

Humour

I told you I was ill.

Spike Milligan's epitaph.

Humour is a great thing. It's not just funny, it's very useful. It creates light where there is fear, is central to relationships, helps us to say the unsayable, breaks tension, humiliates bullies, defines us, creates happiness, raises mood, gives perspective, relaxes, releases endorphins and reduces pain. It is so important that if you have lost it, you need to find it again.

Why we laugh

Just exactly why we laugh is a book in itself. Key themes seem to be a shared perspective, relief that someone shares your experiences, juxtaposed ideas, surprising punchlines, lovable characters, slapstick and catchphrases. It all seems to be about making people feel comfortable and at ease with topics they can relate to, delivered by likeable characters who offer unusual perspectives or quirky mannerisms. Or just say it as it is.

Knowing what makes you laugh is easy. But knowing why can be tricky. In the end, it doesn't matter if you don't know why – but it does matter that you keep enjoying it.

Coping

Finding humour in adversity is used to good effect by people like soldiers and nurses when they need to cope in the face of 'big stuff' where if 'you didn't laugh, you'd cry'. Obviously, they do not always laugh out loud, but their shared humour is bonding and keeps the spirit alive. It helps them to dissociate themselves from upsetting experiences so that they can continue to function.

Change the picture

The way you see things determines how you experience them. So it is important to have ways to frame experiences in a positive or humorous way. One standard piece of advice is that, if someone is annoying you, imagine them naked or on the toilet. A similar but more kindly approach, however, is to think of a funny name for a person or situation that is causing stress.

Janice used to call her thin, stiff leg 'my flamingo leg' to help her to cope. It also helped her talk to her husband about it. This approach does not make the situation hurt less, but it does help her to feel better about it, and that reduces her sadness. By using the term 'flamingo leg', she is normalizing something that might be a taboo.

This kind of humorous reframing helps because the way you think about something affects how you feel, react and behave.

Permission

It is not about just changing the picture, but also about allowing yourself to react in a different way. Daring to see humour in adversity and allowing yourself to have a different reaction is really important. You need to give yourself permission to smile, to say silly things, to massively understate what is happening and to dare to allow a bit of light in.

Large groups of people, like the soldiers and nurses we mentioned above, effectively give each other permission to see the funny side. People with long-term conditions are also an enormous group but do not go around in big groups or wear uniforms that identify them. This means you will have to work on a smaller scale to start exploring humour with close friends and family. Good humour exists when people understand each other, so a shared sense of humour means a shared understanding and vice versa.

Eggshells

There is often a certain kind of walking on eggshells that surrounds chronic pain. No one feels that they have permission to make light of anything, so everything stays dark and heavy. It can also mean that people find it hard to talk to you.

Lots of people say they just want to feel normal, but 'normal' includes humour, and this often seems like a taboo. I suggest that you start walking on your own eggshells and you will lighten your own and everyone else's load. Daring to crack the fragile silence can be a great relief. None of this implies that you do not have pain or a particular condition, it's just that it's better to let a bit of light in. You could say that it is better to 'laugh' than 'cry'.

Losing it (sense of humour failure)

When there is no humour, things seem very serious indeed. In the early stages of any condition, it is probably hard to find any trace of a funny side, but with time, perspectives change and humour can enter if you let it.

Ironically, if someone completely lacks humour, it is hard to take them seriously. And it is easy to lose your sense of humour if you are in pain, stressed, anxious and tired. If you feel physically worn down, you then tend to think down and feel down emotionally. Sensitivity increases, gentle teasing is upsetting, things are taken literally rather than with the usual nuances. As a result, humour flies out of the window.

It is also important to get your sense of humour back because without it you probably do not feel completely yourself and will find it hard to cope with the pain, stress and fatigue. In addition, as others may find it easier to talk openly to you if you maintain your sense of humour, you will be helping them to help you cope.

Wrong(ish) humour

Humour has to be right. If it is forced or inappropriate, it's just not funny. I once attended a laughter therapy session by mistake. The therapist was living up to his title and laughing a lot. In fact, the laughing started on cue just before he came on. He was getting the group to laugh along using his awful 'infectious' laugh, so all of them were laughing and pointing at each other. I didn't laugh.

I squirmed. For me, this was a case of wrong time, wrong place, wrong group.

There is, however, a sort of wisdom in this therapist's approach of using the 'fake it to make it' approach – the idea that if you act in a certain way, you start to feel it. This is certainly true up to a point, and it has its uses. The point here is to be true to yourself; you do not need to laugh to extremes, but maybe you can let yourself laugh or just smile when others are. It is good to let yourself let go a bit and drop your guard.

Finding your humour again

If you are in pain or feeling sad, humour can bounce off you. In many ways, laughing is the very thing you need, but you might have got out of the habit or feel that you are not allowed to find anything funny any more.

Think of humour as being like a muscle that you need to use and 'exercise' again. A good starting point is to dust off some classic comedies, it doesn't matter which. Don't worry if you're not rolling on the floor – just a smile or sense of being among old friends will help.

Pain humour

I'm sticking my neck out here, but it is important to dare to think and talk about a person's difficulties using humour as therapy. The seriousness of the situation is not being ignored, but there is always room for a moment of lightness.

Having a way to refer to difficulties (reframing) helps. It has to be appropriate for you and your situation. Kevin says that when he is feeling odd, he tells his wife that he has 'got the wibbles' (he's a fan of television comedy *Blackadder*); he also calls his crutches Cyril and Cedric. Jane describes her misshaped toe as 'my flipper toe', and Sarah talks about walking like children's cartoon character Pingu the penguin. These are all fantastic ways of using humour to reframe a difficulty in a way that lowers barriers and creates ease around a subject that was previously a no-go area.

Summary

Humour is an important part of life. It is part of all communication and relationships and is a natural coping mechanism that helps us deal with adversity. Humour eventually pops its head up in all situations, but sometimes we can feel that we are not allowed to see the lighter side of events.

I am suggesting, however, that it is vital that you welcome in the lighter side of life. We need to dare to invite it back and start cracking a few more smiles and treading on some of those eggshells. It might feel a bit rebellious or irreverent, but the best laughs always are a bit cheeky. Daring to see the funny side of things is a great coping skill. But it is more than that. It is also part of the joy of living, something that we need so that we can enjoy life despite our difficulties.

Remember, you are in charge. You have the right to be silly, to not take everything seriously, to say the unexpected, to understate wildly, to be ironic, to smile. In fact, you do not just have the right to, you need to. It is all part of life.

In a sentence: it is hard to take seriously a person who takes everything seriously.

16

Others (and yourself)

Fill yourself with yourself and nothing else can get in.

Barefoot Doctor

Dealing with the world is tricky when you are in pain, stressed and vulnerable. It is easy to get it wrong, to misread people and to trip over your own feelings. I thought I would be a bit radical and describe this in terms of bubbles. It gives a different perspective, helping you to step back from difficulties and understand your world better. Personally, I think it's a great way to talk about things.

We all have a 'bubble' around us (Figure 16.1). Some people see this as a bubble of energy, like a force field, while others see it just as a way to describe things. You do not have to believe it actually exists; just use it as a way of thinking about yourself and situations.

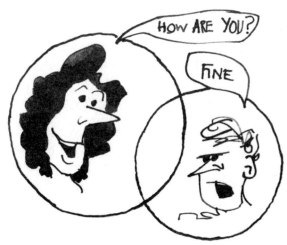

Figure 16.1 You and your bubble

Your bubble contains you and everything about you – your thoughts, your feelings, your everything. When you spend time with other people, your bubbles bump into each other, overlap and merge. Sensitive people can feel someone's mood just by being near their bubble, and couples can find that their bubbles happily merge or start bouncing off each other! When you first come across someone special, you may say 'our eyes met across a crowded room', but maybe it is more accurate to say 'our bubbles merged across a crowded room'. This may be just picking up on body language, but I like to think of it as bubble-sensing.

Some people are described as 'magnetic personalities', and they are the ones with wide bubbles that we all want to be in or near. Conversely, there are other people whose bubbles you would like to avoid. Regardless of this, when you are feeling good your bubble grows, and when you are feeling bad it shrinks. You will particularly notice this on a difficult day when you need more personal space, because your shrunken bubble makes you feel more vulnerable to the presence of others, so you want to make sure they are further away.

On a big bubble day, you will feel safer, so you will be less sensitive to the world. This means that you will be able to enjoy a bit of give and take or a joke and see things relatively positively. In effect, anything 'bad' tends to bounce off your bubble. But on a small bubble day, the world seems to be an unpleasant place where everyone seems to say the wrong thing to you. Anything potentially critical or annoying that would normally just bounce off you tends to get through into the bubble and upset you.

Emotional GORE-TEX®

Unfortunately, that bubble sometimes behaves like a form of really inefficient GORE-TEX® – the clothing material that usually acts to deflect rain and let moisture out. If the bubble is small, it lets in criticism and keeps out compliments. This is known as minimizing (the good) and maximizing (the bad).

We have bad GORE-TEX®, or small bubble, days when we are stressed, tired or in pain. In these circumstances, there is no energy left for working out subtleties, and we tend to go into alert mode because we feel vulnerable. And then we can easily misunderstand what people mean, often taking things literally or negatively. 'You look well' might be read as 'There's nothing wrong with you, is there?' 'How are you?' could be taken literally and met with 'Isn't it obvious?' rather than as the 'Hello' it really means.

Awareness

The main 'tool' for improvement is awareness. This does not sound like an amazing or exciting technique, but just knowing that you are having a small, or bad, bubble day is useful because you then know in advance that the world will seem far worse than it actually is. You will also know that you should keep an eye on yourself to spot when you are taking things too literally or negatively, or simply realize that you are just plain grumpy. Remember that it is a bad bubble day for you, not a bad day everywhere.

Certain clues can indicate that a bad bubble day is about to happen, even if it is not obvious at first. The main culprits for shrinking bubbles are:

- lack of sleep
- pain
- stress
- worry.

Don't beat yourself up about a small bubble day, but realize that you will be seeing the world as worse than it really is. You will probably feel more threatened and may snap at people for saying the 'wrong' things. You may also think more negative thoughts about yourself and your situation, perhaps that your pain will never change and that things will only get worse.

NAGs come out to play

When bubbles shrink, NAGs – the negative automatic thoughts that we met in Chapter 11 – come out to play. NAGs deflate bubbles very easily, so you need to be aware of the mischief they can create.

A NAG is just what it sounds like, a persistent, annoying, unhelpful criticism, or 'negative automatic garbage'. It is like someone is telling you that you should expect the worst, you're not good enough, you should always do better, you don't belong, you're a bad person, you should worry, you should always be winning. But it is not someone else saying these things, it's you yourself, and you often do not know you are doing it. So it will seem like you really are a bad person and that the world genuinely is an awful place. What is actually happening is that you are just playing an old thoughts record. Everyone has this kind of 'self-talk', and it always comes to the surface when we are under pressure.

It is hard to get rid of NAGs because they often date from childhood, but you can become aware of what they are so that you can remind yourself you are seeing the world through an unhelpful set of NAG glasses. Going further, you can start to challenge those NAGs and prove to yourself that they no longer belong, or just see them for what they are – outdated ideas that no longer belong in your bubble.

Managing your bubble

Allow yourself to have a bad bubble day

It is fine to have a bad bubble day. These things happen, and they happen more often if you have a mountain on your plate. So don't make things even worse by feeling bad for feeling bad. It's OK not to be OK.

Relax more

Calmer people have bigger bubbles. So regular relaxation, or just time out doing nothing much, is important. This of course needs to be balanced by other periods of work, which can be paid or unpaid.

Refocus

Paying attention to difficulties makes bubbles shrink, so if you lose yourself in something you find important and you are good at, such as a hobby or project, your bubble will grow again. Some people call this sort of losing yourself 'Flow'.

First aid for your bubble

When your bubble shrinks, pump it up a bit by stopping what you are doing and concentrating on breathing slowly for ten breaths.

Affirmations

The opposite of a NAG is a positive affirmation or statement. Having a good affirmation helps to reassure you and to argue against the false logic of your NAGs. Keep saying to yourself what you need to hear. Here are some you could adopt.

- 'I'm good enough for me.'
- 'I'm doing my best and that's as much as I can do.'
- 'Things will improve.'
- 'This too shall pass.'
- 'Every day, in every way, I am getting better and better' (a famous mantra from French psychologist Émile Coué).

Visualize

This sounds a bit subtle, but visualization works if you are good with images. Try seeing or imagining a protective bubble around you. What is its colour? What are its other qualities, such as shape and thickness? Is it shiny or matt? Is it moving or is it still? You could also practically assess your bubble by being aware of how near people are before they make you feel twitchy.

See it touching things, such as the walls or other people, and then try to imagine growing it out from you. Grow it out to fill your room, your house, your town and out to the horizon. Get it to fill any place or situation that you are anxious about, so that when you go there, you have 'been' there before. I used to do this every morning in the car before starting sessions with a highly bubble-shrinking client.

Mingle

Other people with small bubbles may drain you, but being on your own might shrink your bubble more. Therefore, it helps to get out and socialize with people who make your bubble grow.

Talk in bubble terms

It's useful to talk to others who will understand the bubble idea. It is a way of talking about yourself in general terms rather than needing to go into detail that you do not want to share or may not even be aware of. A discussion about bubbles can lead to understanding and a focus on what to do to make your bubble grow. Indeed, just talking makes it grow as long as you are talking to the right sort of person.

Others' bubbles

Whenever someone upsets you, think about the interaction between your bubbles. What's in yours, what's in theirs? This is another version of the saying 'Is it my rubbish or theirs?' Do you have a sensitivity, a doubt or a NAG in your bubble that is being prodded? Or do they have something in theirs that is causing them to affect you? Are you bouncing off each other?

Understanding what is in others' bubbles allows you to understand them as people, and know what they mean and how to communicate with them. This is the basis for successful communication and ties in with the idea 'seek first to understand and then to be understood'.

Boundaries

Other people may come wandering into our bubbles without our permission. This is known as a boundary issue. If you think people are coming in and draining you, it is important to be aware of what is or is not appropriate for you and let others know. Although most people will have a natural sense of boundaries, they sometimes need to be reminded – for the sake of your bubble.

Bubble vampires

Some people seek to pump up their own bubbles by unconsciously sucking energy out of yours. They might do it through their behaviour or by what they say. A good example is the person who always puts you down, or an acquaintance who makes you feel exhausted for no obvious reason.

Listen and reason with yourself

If your bubble is small, you need to really listen to what people say rather than instantly jumping in to react against it. A small bubble makes it hard to think in a straight line, so consider the logic of your reactions. Do people really mean what you think you are hearing?

Sleep

A good night's sleep is important (see Chapter 7). If you do not sleep well, find a good relaxation technique to practise (some suggestions are given in Chapter 6) and look into the topic of 'sleep hygiene' to promote better sleep.

Confidence

To paraphrase the quote at the start of the chapter, 'If you fill your bubble with yourself, nothing can get in.' This means being yourself with pride and confidence, and being sure about yourself. Dispelling self-doubt is great for the size of your bubble.

Summary

Talking about bubbles is a fun, light-hearted way to raise awareness of many of the issues that are important in managing health and improving well-being. It is a useful approach because we can talk in general terms without having to dig up all sorts of painful issues that we might not want to share. If you can be self-aware enough to recognize a 'bad bubble day', you are already one step removed from feeling completely miserable. This kind of awareness means that you can try to see through the fog created by stress, pain and fatigue. It also encourages you to start talking about what you should be doing to make that bubble grow.

17

Punk pain management

I'm a real rebel with a cause.

Nina Simone

When I was a student there were lots of trendy types who thought they were rebellious. In those days, it meant wearing badges that showed your political allegiances, having wild hair, sticking a Che Guevara poster on your bedroom wall, smoking roll-ups and listening to punk music. Ironically, trying to look different produced armies of 'alternative' people who all looked the same. Obviously, the rebellion was all part of growing up and raging against the 'machine' at a stage in life when it did not really matter.

On reflection it was all quite funny. There was even an Anarchy Society whose members weren't alive to the irony of their group, with its committee and rules. Theirs was a sort of empty, self-indulgent rebellion based on a no-risk backlash against nice middle-class comforts. And on the whole the rebellion burnt itself out when it came to the graduate jobs fair. In those days, about a third of all graduates were recruited to become accountants, which wasn't very punk!

Despite all the strange hair, ripped jeans and badges, being a rebel is often a good thing because it is all about finding out who you are and daring to question the status quo. Most children rebel against their parents, no matter how lovely they are. I had a friend whose parents were very trendy alternative types and his rebellion was to become incredibly conventional. So there is rebellion in everyone no matter what direction it goes in. And thankfully, you don't have to look rebellious to be rebellious.

In pain management, you might need to become a proper rebel, a pain management punk. Rest assured, you don't have to do the hair thing and you can still like Abba. But what you *do* need to do is question the rules and expectations that might be confining and defining you.

Being a rebel might sound like behaving badly, but when you think about it, it makes perfect sense. With chronic pain, it is easy to feel like an 'outsider' and a lot of anguish occurs when we try to stay 'normal' and conform to what convention says we should do. This is fine if we are capable of doing it, and happy to do so, but what if it causes unnecessary distress? If you are upset by what convention 'says', you are right to be defiant and fight back. You are right to say, 'I'm not prepared to tolerate this.'

A major issue for many is concern about what others will say and think about them. The social stigma associated with unseen conditions such as chronic pain means that we have to work extra hard to regain our dignity and confidence, dare to be ourselves and learn to ignore critics. We could plod away trying to carefully rebuild things, but sometimes you need to let rip and tap into a bit of punk power.

As we said in Chapter 2, there are two defining issues in pain management: stress and overdoing things. These are largely created by the battle to come to terms with a change in what you can do and the wish to feel accepted and normal. A big part of the battle is trying to maintain standards and live up to expectations. These are both your own standards and what you think other people expect of you. If you are stressed, this all becomes overwhelming, and it is common to experience enormous anxiety and guilt. It goes without saying that pain plus anxiety and guilt is a nasty cocktail. And punks don't drink cocktails!

Rules

We all have rules that guide us, and rules are, up to a point, a good thing. But what if those rules are unhelpful? What if they are based on a situation and result from a time that did not consider health issues as part of your personal equation? What if the rules you have are making you miserable? What if they are unfair? What if they are now wrong?

Before going any further, I need to say that when we are struggling in life, reverting to the familiar 'rules' is a natural reflex. Familiarity and certainty are attractive, but they can be a 'honey trap' that keeps us stuck. People can become 'comfortably uncomfortable'. Similarly, hiding away so that you prevent what you think will be public censure can be a safe approach – but a miserable one.

In pain management, we need to question the 'rules' and ask 'What about me?' Spiky-haired punk Toyah once sang that she 'wanted to be free' and tautologically she also 'wanted to be me', and that's worth remembering. Some of the 'rules' that are worth shaking a fist at might seem trivial, but if left unchallenged they cause difficulties when you cannot reach the standard written in your own rule book.

So ask yourself these punk questions.

- 'Who says?'
- 'Why?'
- 'What would happen if I didn't follow the rules?'

And shake a fist at some of the following ideas. I know it's not very punky, but these rules do literally end up ruling our lives in a bad way, so it is very important that we loosen their grip on us.

- 'I have to maintain standards regardless.'
- 'My worth comes only from what I do.'
- 'If I start a job, I have to finish it.'
- 'I must keep everybody happy.'
- 'I have to be on the go all the time.'
- 'My needs come last.'
- 'I can't ask for help.'
- 'Health is only sorted by doctors.'
- 'I need approval or permission to do what I need to do.'
- 'I can't upset the apple cart.'
- 'No one will understand.'
- 'No one cares.'
- 'If I accept my condition, it means that I've given up.'
- 'It's better to stick with what I know.'
- 'I must work hard regardless.'

I'm sure you have identified a few that you could do with rebelling against. Or at least adjusting a bit. At this stage, it's easy to say 'yes, but' – but you could also dare to think otherwise. Sometimes we do not realize how things are affecting us. And if you feel that it is too difficult to change right now, it is helpful to become aware of just how much a rule might be affecting you. Armed with that information, you might find yourself quietly rebelling and possibly releasing some anger, especially if these rules are making you feel unnecessarily bad about yourself.

Use your anger positively

Most punks always seemed to be a bit angry but I never dared to ask what exactly they were angry about!

John Lydon (aka Johnny Rotten), of Sex Pistols and Public Image Ltd fame, sang about anger being an energy, and it certainly is. Anger involves an enormous amount of energy that helps and urges us to deal with what is wrong or threatening us. The trouble is that being angry in the long term wears people out.

Many people with chronic pain will admit to at least some anger. That anger might be against the medical profession, against people who do not understand or simply about what has happened. In addition, being in pain makes us feel more vulnerable, so we can be generally angry as an unconscious defence mechanism to scare people off so they don't dare challenge us.

The trouble with anger is that, if you do not use it to do something useful to deal with threats, it becomes a kind of empty anger that can just beat you up and scare your family and friends away. It can also make you fight the wrong battles, such as forcing yourself on to do more than the pain is actually allowing you to do. Above all, anger is a stress state that will wind up pain and make it harder to see the wood for the trees.

When they need to deal with change, people are often angry about what has happened but continue to 'toe the line' and keep trying to maintain values and fit in; in this way, they want to feel normal. But the process of doing this leads to more frustration and anger instead. So how about getting angry for a bit and recognizing that the rules causing your misery need to be overturned? And that you do not need permission to look after yourself. You especially do not need permission from people who don't or won't understand.

Punk rules

If you fillet out the good stuff and forget the fashion statements, there's a lot to be said about a genuine 'punk' approach to pain management. It is surprisingly in tune with the personal rebellion you need to make to break free and move on.

In a few lines, my own version of pain management punk goes as follows.

- Dare to be honest with yourself and see things clearly.
- When you see things clearly, you will probably get angry – so put that anger into action. That anger will help you to overcome your 'yes, buts'.
- Don't sit on your anger. Remember it's an energy, so use it.
- Stop not wanting to offend people who are offending you with their attitudes.
- Express yourself.
- Be intolerant of what is confining you against your will or best interests.
- Recognize your emotions, understand what they are saying to you and act on them in ways that help you.
- Value yourself.
- Fight to be yourself and improve your life.
- Stick up for the truth.
- You only need permission from yourself.
- You are your own authority.
- Don't be defined by stereotypes (whether described by yourself or someone else).
- Dare to challenge convention and complacency.
- Rip up the rule book, or at least shake a fist at it.
- Express your emotions and don't hold them all in.
- If you know you are right and know it will be good for you – act on it.
- Don't be ruled by others.
- Sod the critics!

Summary

As you can see, this is all a bit radical, but that is what rebellion is. If you are stuck, it is vital to adopt the essence of the punk approach. As an older wiser type, you will be able to take these fierce ideas and apply them with subtlety to create the changes you need to unstick yourself and move on to enjoy a better life. Ultimately, it is about daring to be yourself again – and that is a very good thing indeed.

It's time to start spiking your metaphorical hair, saying Boo! to the world and yourself, and start rebelling a bit.

References and further reading

Burch, Vidyamala and Penman, Danny (2013) *Mindfulness for Health*. London: Piatkus.

Butler, David and Moseley, Lorimer (2013) *Explain Pain* (2nd edn). Alton, Hampshire: NOI.

Cantopher, Tim (2003) *Depressive Illness: The curse of the strong*. London: Sheldon Press.

Cole, Frances (2012) *Overcoming Chronic Pain*. London: Robinson.

Eccleston, Christopher (2011) 'A normal psychology of pain', *Pain Management*, 1:399–403.

Eccleston, Christopher (2016) *Embodied: The psychology of physical sensation*. Oxford: Oxford University Press.

Enders, Giulia (2015) *Gut*. London: Scribe UK.

Gilbert, Paul (2009) *Overcoming Depression*. London: Robinson.

Haines, Steven C. (2015) *Pain is Really Strange*. London: Singing Dragon.

Hayes, Steven (2005) *Get Out of Your Mind and into Your Life*. Oakland, CA: New Harbinger.

Hoff, Benjamin (1982) *The Tao of Pooh*. London: Egmont.

Melzack, Ronald and Wall, Patrick D. (1996) *The Challenge of Pain*. Harmondsworth, Middlesex: Penguin.

Mosley, Michael (2017) *The Clever Guts Diet*. London: Short Books.

Roet, Brian (1996) *All in the Mind?* London: Vermilion.

Roet, Brian (1986) *Hypnosis: A gateway to better health*. London: J. M. Dent.

Saplosky, Robert (2004) *Why Zebras Don't Get Ulcers* (revised edn). New York: St Martin's Press.

Shone, Neville (2008) *The Chronic Pain Diet Book*. London: Sheldon Press.

Sizer, Phil (n.d.). *Simple Relaxation* (CD). See www.painassociation.com.

Tolle, Eckhart (2001) *The Power of Now: A guide to spiritual enlightenment*. London: Yellow Kite.

Walker, Matthew (2017) *Why We Sleep*. Harmondsworth, Middlesex: Penguin.

Wax, Ruby (2013) *Sane New World: Taming the mind*. London: Hodder & Stoughton.

Index